G000138011

WEIGHT LOSS
WINNERS
&
DIETING
DOWNFALLS

Alyssa Burns-Hill, PhD

Bio-Vitality.com

Published by Bio-Vitality
P O Box 493
Guernsey
UK

ISBN - 978-1-906446-99-4

First Edition

DEDICATION

For Weight Loss Winners Everywhere!

CONTENTS

PREFACE

Diets have been around for years and have a self-depriving overtone to them, which can be a hard nut to crack if you're feeling tired, can't sleep and are pretty low in mood. You're probably doomed to failure before you begin. Wouldn't it be good if you could work in better harmony with your body? Wouldn't it be good if eating wasn't such a battle between desire and need? These ideas can become a reality through working *with* your hormones instead of being on a roller-coaster fuelled by hormonal excesses and deficiencies.

Over the years many people have come into my clinic telling me about the problems they have experienced when they try to lose weight. Some of them have been to their doctor in the hope that they have a thyroid problem that will explain why the weight isn't shifting as fast as it could be. For those of you who do manage to have their thyroid hormone levels checked there is usually a 'normal' response from your doctor, which can be very disappointing. However, hormones aren't that simplistic, there are many hormone imbalances that can seriously impact your ability to lose weight and your success at keeping it off. For the people who work with me to understand and balance their hormones more naturally they find that by doing very little they can lose between 2–7lbs (on average) within 6 weeks without dieting or changing what they're doing.

So what's going on?

Awareness and understanding of what you're doing and why you're doing it can make a profound difference to how you eat and how you live your life. You could be making easy minor adjustments that have major impacts in terms of weight loss and energy levels. Does that sound unbelievable? Here are some testimonial examples from clients who worked on understanding and balancing their hormones as well as following a healthier eating plan …

Sandie, from Greece, was pleased how things worked out for her:

I'm writing to inform you that I am feeling very much improved. My memory has improved, my general mood has uplifted and I no longer am depressed. I have lost weight, but most importantly, that bulge around the hips has disappeared allowing the feminine curves to re-appear.

Keri, from the UK, *reported:*

Everything seems to be kicking in now, I'm losing weight and feel more energetic. Can still be a bit tired at times especially in the morning waking up but is definitely getting better, so much so I have started doing some yoga in the mornings. I've been following a really healthy way of eating and weight is coming down slowly but the fact it's coming down is brilliant.

Jackie, from UK, also experienced a big shift in her success levels:

I must say I am feeling great about the new regime and have lost 8 kg (over 17 lbs).

My clinics are busy with people who often include their weight as problematic, but generally just want to feel better about themselves. Often I'm told that they feel that they're not the person they used to be and this contributes to their need to comfort eat. I help them to find their 'old self' once more, which helps them to feel more in control of their life, so that they can make the changes that need to be made and maintain them on a sustainable basis. It's a great process that's a privilege to witness.

My wish is that you find the information in this book truly empowering, leading you to better health and wellbeing that brings you weight loss as a satisfying side effect.

INTRODUCTION

When it comes to weight loss, hormones can be both your friends and your enemies. This book is about how you back your winners in order to defeat your enemies and make your weight management frustrations a thing of the past.

There are some points I'd like to make clear so that we are all on the same page: this is not a complex, 'sciencey' and theoretical book. It's a practical, easy-to-understand approach that you can use to achieve real and lasting results.

This is not another calorie-controlled diet fad. It's about using tips and tricks to:

Maximise your metabolism;

Ease the pressure on your willpower;

> Make better decisions about what you eat and when;
>
> Nourish the body and feed the soul (a little of what you fancy does you good).

I don't believe in diet sheets, diet pills or products – there is always a compromise ...

> Following strict regimes is stressful and highlights hard or unpleasant choices;
>
> Negative health consequences - don't use diet pills or lo-cal, artificially sweetened options, you're not cheating the system but you are cheating your health;
>
> Negative financial consequences on your wallet as you radically change your grocery shopping.

This book is about a more person-centred perspective, using scientific understanding that will make sense to you and provide you with a cost effective, health promoting SIMPLE and SUSTAINABLE approach to losing and maintaining your weight - no matter what sort of diet regime you choose to follow.

Alongside learning about weight loss you will be able to:

> Reduce your risk of diabetes, heart disease and

cancer;

Reduce your risk, or experience, of depression, anxiety, stress, irritability, mood swings, sugar cravings, low energy and more ...;

Improve your sleep so that you wake up feeling rested and not reaching for coffee and a pastry (or high sugar cereal) to get you going;

Be motivated to exercise in a way that works for you and in a way that helps you to feel better.

Yes, you truly can learn all these things and No, they are not complicated or time consuming or expensive.

DIETING: IT'S NOT ABOUT WILLPOWER

Losing weight is not simply a mathematical outcome.

Don't be fooled by weight loss regimes that want to make you believe that the problem is purely a mathematical equation that goes like this:

less calories in against more energy expended = weight loss.

Well, yes, to a point this does work for some people in the short term, but once you go back to eating normally, the weight often piles back on, sometimes faster than ever.

The weight loss picture is more complex than that because you're a person not a machine. Surprising new research has revealed that the average Brit might spend more than half of the year on a diet and three quarters of us are unhappy with our weight. Dieting is a time-consuming and a miserable process that often has poor results or results that don't last.

It's generally thought that dieting or losing weight is about willpower – the ability to say 'No' to food. Anyone who can't say no and moderate their intake is just going to get fatter and fatter and we should judge them harshly, right? Well, no, it's not fair to be so harsh because we are all at the mercy of our hormones and they can, and will, sabotage your efforts or hijack your willpower. This can leave you:

Feeling anxious or stressed and seeking solace (*food*);
Feeling depressed and seeking comfort (*food*);
Feeling tired and seeking energy (*food*);
Having cravings that need satisfying (*food*);
Not losing weight despite cutting your consumption down to say 1,000 carefully counted calories per day, which leaves you feeling depressed and seeking comfort (*food*)!

Let alone thinking about where hunger comes into the day, it can be a real merry-go-round.

There are also other factors that may be holding you back:

Bad habits;
Lack of exercise;
Too many choices;
The excuse of getting older;
Poor self-image and lack of belief that you can do it;
Too much reliance on packaged foods.

So, all in all, you can see that the human mechanics of losing weight are not just about calorie restriction.

At this point I don't want you to feel that your task is insurmountable and that you are likely to be continuing a lifetime of losing a few pounds only to put them on again and more besides, which is the typical scenario. Dieting and losing weight has unseen elements that can be pulling your strings and affecting your:

Determination;
Motivation;
Metabolism; and, ultimately
Success in the short term through to the long term.

Hormone Buttons and Self-Medication

The truth is that most of the problems you are going to encounter in your weight loss nightmare are hormonal. So, whilst it is all about you, it's not all in your control if you are constantly pressing the wrong 'hormone buttons'. For example:

a hormone button that squashes your metabolism,

which means less or no weight loss, low energy, fatigue and constipation. (No fun when you're dieting!);

or,

a hormone button that means that you crave sugar like crazy and your willpower at 3.30 in the afternoon hits rock bottom as your colleague offers you your usual chocolate bar/doughnut/biscuit to keep you going. Your body has come to expect this little mid-afternoon pick-me-up, so what's a girl or guy to do?

(Saying no can be especially difficult if you've had a stressful day or, if you're a girl, if it's before your period! I'll explain more on this later.)

Another area of constant frustration can be exercise, which often becomes a problem because of time pressures and lack of energy. It's an easy sacrifice because you can blame work, lack of sleep, or even the children or your partner. It's much easier to go home, have supper and a beer, or glass of wine, to unwind after a tiring and stressful day in order to recuperate enough for the next day. But that's more self-medication just like the sugar hit at 3.30 in the afternoon mentioned above. Self-medication is when you self-prescribe an off-the-shelf remedy for the rubbish way you're feeling and here are some common examples:

Feeling tired and sluggish in the morning – coffee/tea (hit of caffeine - stimulant);

Needing energy to go with that jolt of caffeine – simple carb cereal, a pastry or toast and jam (sugar – stimulant);

Energy slump mid-afternoon – chocolate, cake or a biscuit (sugar - stimulant);

The end of another stressful week and you made it! – Friday after work drink (alcohol – relaxant but this will cause carb cravings);

Keeping your energy and mental sharpness up to meet a looming deadline? – coffee, tea or even a cola (caffeine and sugar – stimulant);

Feeling low, or lonely or had an argument? – cake, or cereal or chocolate (carbs boost serotonin production – serotonin is your 'happy' hormone, and/or oxytocin - your 'hug' hormone).

Whether you use alcohol, sugar, caffeine, prescription or over-the-counter drugs, your body is being medicated to unwind, produce energy, feel less anxious or less pain, or wake up! Your hormones are calling you and begging for your attention! We often don't realise that we're self-medicating to feel better and that you'll be reaching for your chosen medication without thinking because it's your body screaming at you, "Gimme".

These are all things you will have learned as you grew up in family life, socially or even because of tv programmes or adverts. You saw the behaviour or food, tried it and experienced the effect. Your body experienced a response, "aaah, that's better," and you're hooked.

WHY HORMONES ARE IMPORTANT IN WEIGHT MANAGEMENT

How Hormones Affect Us

In my experience the majority of people think that hormones are all about women's problems: the menstrual cycle, pregnancy, fertility and menopause. But hormones are the body's chemical messengers that affect us *all* physically, mentally and emotionally. Here are a few examples of the influences of hormones for men and women:

energy levels, mood swings, dealing with stress, ability to think properly, memory, weight management, libido, weight distribution, sleep, aches and pains, connection with people, feelings of depression and anxiety, feeling calm, feeling loved and nurtured, etc, etc.

As chemical messengers, hormones are released or secreted by glands into the blood stream or nervous system where they travel to their target tissues. There are receptors in the target tissue and these receptors are just like docking stations that each individual hormone recognises and can connect with, but there are many factors that can interfere with their *availability* to dock and their *ability* to dock. These are two reasons why hormone health can be complex and why it's more than being about lab results reflecting absolute and accurate data about hormone levels and function. There are many well documented signs and symptoms that will accurately reflect an individual's hormone imbalance experience. So, with hormones, reading between the lines and joining the dots is vital to having an accurate reflection and interpretation of what the person is experiencing.

I hope you can now begin to see the importance and diversity of these very powerful body chemicals, but let's concentrate on weight management factors and go a little deeper.

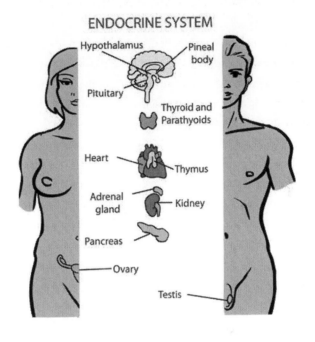

ENDOCRINE SYSTEM

Hypothalamus
Pineal body
Pituitary
Thyroid and Parathyoids
Heart
Thymus
Adrenal gland
Kidney
Pancreas
Ovary
Testis

We're not going to concentrate on what some people think are the important hormones when it comes to weight loss: ghrelin and leptin, the hunger and satiety (feeling full) hormones. Why? Because that assumes an isolated cause and effect relationship with weight management problems. We're going to think of you as a person with a number of factors coming into play instead of an individual at the mercy of two isolated hormones that are directly linked with rather obvious factors in weight management.

Your Hormone's Operate in a System - Not in Isolation

Your hormonal chain of command starts in your brain's limbic system or, your emotional centre. Without going into too much detail, this is why your hormone levels can be directed by your mental and emotional responses, which means that although your hormones can control you and your responses, you and your responses will also affect your hormones! It's a bit of a chicken and egg conundrum, which is where mind-body medicine comes in. Mind-body medicine is about how connected and responsive your body's reactions are to your personal experience of life and vice versa. Let me give you an example: if you are stressed and not sleeping very well someone at work might irritate you and put you in a bad mood. This will trigger your Hypothalamus in your limbic centre to send out CRF (Corticotropin Releasing Factor), which goes to the Pituitary (in your brain and is considered to be your hormonal control centre) to send out ACTH (Adrenocorticotropic Hormone) to stimulate the Adrenal gland to secrete more Cortisol, your stress hormone. This chain of events means that your blood sugar will drop, causing more irritability and fatigue, and then you might want to reach for comfort food and energy (sugar)! The body's drive for this is multi-factored – the comfort food will give your energy levels a boost and it will also boost your level of serotonin (your 'happy' hormone), which will give your mood a lift. This will help you to feel less stressed and irritable, which will mean that the stimulus for more cortisol will drop and you won't feel so agitated. If you reach for a cream cake or pastry (with sugar *and* fat) you'll also get a good hit of oxytocin, which will calm you and give you a feeling of 'there, there, there.'

Is this a scenario that you can relate to? This is exactly why losing weight and making good eating decisions is more complex than sticking to a calorie controlled diet sheet.

Key Glands and Hormones that May be Affecting Your Weight

The Thyroid

The Thyroid Gland is probably most commonly complained about when a person has weight management problems that they believe cannot be explained otherwise.

The thyroid gland question is a tricky one because we expect our doctor to be able to diagnose and treat it, but the problem is not always medical and disease-focused. Hormones from the gland have to function and connect in order to be successful in their task, for example, thyroid hormone function can be interfered with by stress, other hormone imbalances, nutritional deficiencies and toxicities. These are probably areas best sorted out and supported by more natural and holistic means rather than drugs or hormone supplementation because it's all about creating a healthy environment for hormones to function in.

So what have we established here?

Thyroid-related problems can be present without having a failing gland and this can mean that you experience many, or some, of the symptoms related to an under-active thyroid. These problems can include generalised weight gain, depression, foggy thinking and fatigue. Anyone suffering with these problems will have a compromised attitude towards food and making good choices, let alone finding willpower to diet if they are feeling down and have found that calorie restriction diets can be desperately unfruitful. I recall working with a woman who came to me in desperation and tears. She had worked so hard to lose weight and was weighing her food and conscientiously counting the calories of every morsel that passed her lips and she had done this for quite some time, yet she still wasn't losing weight. She was convinced that she had a thyroid problem and on her last visit to her doctor she told him that she had cut her calorie consumption down to 800 per day and was still not losing weight. She pleaded with him to do another thyroid test that had previously come back in 'normal' range. His response was a definite 'No', and that she should just eat less! This woman worked with me and we discovered that she was not converting her T4 (the main thyroid hormone secreted by the gland) to T3 (the main thyroid hormone that does most of the work) properly due to high stress and nutritional deficiencies. We worked on her situation and as her mood lifted, so did her stress; her weight started to fall away and she had more energy to cope.

Some hormones in the thyroid pathway: Thyroid Stimulating Hormone (TSH) tells the thyroid to secrete Thyroxine (T4), T4 must be converted to T3 (Thyronine) in order for your body to have effective levels of thyroid hormone to work with.

The Adrenals

Your adrenal glands sit atop your kidneys and adrenal health is an area that medicine often fails to recognise the importance of in a world filled with stressed out people.

Cortisol and DHEAS are the main stress hormones secreted by the outer part of the adrenal (Adrenal Cortex) in response to stress. Adrenaline and noradrenaline are secreted by the inner part of the adrenal (Adrenal Medulla) into the nervous system and these hormones are recognised as your 'fight or flight' hormones.

Misunderstood and Under-Estimated

Stress is a very misunderstood concept that people

believe is always related to current external life events and is generally judged on a subjective scale. My stress is not as bad as his stress; or, perhaps it's a case of self-talk telling you that you have a good life and nothing to be stressed about. Because of media exposure to the term we all accept a certain amount of stress as part of our lives, but if it goes too far it can end up being diagnosed as a mental health problem, or, have devastating effects on your physical health.

Medicine looks at your adrenals from a disease point of view and a simplification of the scenario is what I shall call an Adrenal Stress Continuum. Medicine considers that 'normal' cortisol adrenal function is anything more than Addison's Disease and less than Cushing's Syndrome, which leaves a huge range of what is considered to be 'normal' (see the diagram below). However, the stresses you are exposed to in your life take their toll on your adrenals either acutely (for a short time) or chronically (for a long time), which may affect the continuing ability of your adrenals to respond effectively to the demands made upon them. When this happens your health and wellbeing can be significantly undermined on a day by day basis.

Adrenal Stress Continuum

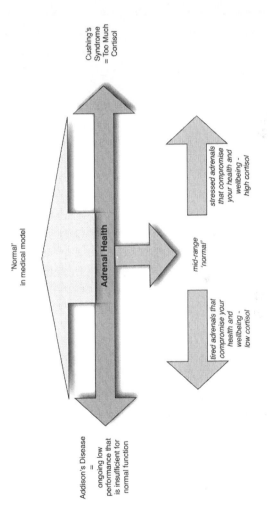

'Normal' in medical model

Addison's Disease = ongoing low performance that is insufficient for normal function

Adrenal Health

tired adrenals that compromise your health and wellbeing - low cortisol

mid-range 'normal'

stressed adrenals that compromise your health and wellbeing - high cortisol

Cushing's Syndrome = Too Much Cortisol

Your responses to certain situations will depend on your background of stress – what you have experienced previously will play a large part in your perception of the potentially stressful event as well as your adrenal capacity to respond to it. If you had a negative or difficult experience or outcome previously it will ramp up feelings of anxiety, irritability, or lack of being able to think properly. The situation might overwhelm you because your adrenals are tired or it might send you into a rage because your adrenals are stressed. Your reactions to stress can change as you get older because of your stress history and your adrenal capacity to respond. Little things that you used to deal with easily can become overwhelming and send you into a little crumpled heap. When you reflect later you may wonder why this happens because it's not you. Adrenal capacity will dramatically affect your mental and emotional state, creating a poor sense of wellbeing and a loss in self-confidence that can be very worrying.

Some hormones in the adrenal pathway: Adreno-corticotropin hormone (ACTH) from the pituitary gland tells the outer part of the adrenal gland to secrete Cortisol and DHEAS (Dehydroepiandrosterone) in order for your body to have effective levels of hormones to deal with stress as well as a lot of other important functions such as: blood sugar regulation, blood pressure and immune response.

The Pancreas

The Pancreas secretes insulin, your blood glucose (sugar) *absorbing* hormone from the *beta* cells of the islets of Langerhans. The *alpha* cells secrete the blood glucose *generating* hormone, glucagon. Together these hormones form the body's feedback system that regulates the amount of glucose in your blood.

Glucagon, is insulin's partner hormone and breaks down stored fats to use as an energy source. Eating low carbohydrate and protein rich meals can help to boost your glucagon levels, which will assist in weight loss aims. This type of diet can also help to support insulin sensitivity, the opposite of insulin resistance. When your cells become resistant to the effects of insulin (because of over exposure) it is known as insulin resistance, or pre-diabetes, which can lead to Type II diabetes requiring medication, or, if you deal with the diet and lifestyle issues causing the insulin resistance it can be reversed if it has not gone too far.

The problem of diabetes is a growing concern, especially as its prevalence in younger people has seen the sharpest rise in the last twenty years according to research done at Cardiff University (2013).

Understanding the mechanisms involved in creating a potentially diabetic situation is important information to arm yourself with and there are two things that will dramatically increase your risk: sugar/carbohydrate rich diet and stress, or rather, the influence of cortisol, your stress hormone.

The Carb Yo-Yo Routine

As you consume foods in the simple carbohydrate food group, such as potato, pasta, bread, cakes, biscuits, sweets, etc, they are absorbed and metabolised into the body very quickly and become blood glucose (sugar). Rising levels of blood glucose will trigger the secretion of insulin. If you keep filling up on simple carbs your body keeps pushing out blood glucose and keeps releasing insulin to control it. If this process happens too often and with too much sugar in your diet, your cells will start to become resistant to insulin through over-exposure.

Signs that are linked to consistently high levels of insulin are: fluctuating blood pressure, sugar cravings, weight gain around the middle, irritability, acne, memory and concentration problems, tiredness and depression.

Good tests to do to find out how your insulin and blood sugar levels are doing are:

HbA1c – most doctors are able to do this test and it should be between 4 – 5.9%. This test is far more helpful than a spot glucose test as it provides an average of your blood sugar levels over the last 3 months.

Fasting Insulin – is the most direct method of checking your level and unfortunately this is a test that is not usually available on the NHS in the UK, but may be available in other countries. (It is a test that is available on my website. Both insulin and HbA1C can be tested as part of the Diabetes Profile.)

Your Metabolic Fire

There's a metaphor that I like to use that makes it easy to remember better sources of energy and understand the game you're playing with your body in the Carb Yo-Yo Routine.

If you imagine that your metabolism is a fire, so you have your metabolic fire that needs feeding to keep your energy levels up. If you put simple carbs on your fire it's like putting paper on a real fire …. Whoosh, whoosh, big heat then it's gone. This is just like the effect of simple carbs on your body – sudden release of glucose into the blood stream giving lots of energy and then gone in a big drop, leaving you feeling empty and irritable. However, if you put protein on your metabolic fire it's like putting a log on a real fire. It's a slow burn, giving a slower release of glucose into the bloodstream, which will give you a much more even feeling of energy that will sustain you for longer, and this will help you to maintain a more stable blood sugar and energy levels for body and mind, helping you to make better choices when it comes to your meals or snacks because you won't feel so desperate and irritable.

Stress

We're back to the adrenals again! But this time I want to concentrate more on the impact of higher cortisol levels on insulin. As we know stress causes higher levels of cortisol in the blood stream and on a sustained basis this can really mess around with your blood glucose levels because cortisol will block insulin from its receptors (docking stations). If insulin is not connecting and ushering in the blood glucose into the cells, it will get higher and higher as insulin resistance becomes more and more of a problem over time. The signals your body sends out when this is happing are likely to cause sugar cravings because your body thinks that it's starving because it can't get access to the blood glucose that's there.

This is also the time when cortisol will mobilise

cholesterol-like fats, called triglycerides, to storage in the tummy area. This is fat storage that's not superficial, it's laid down deep in the abdomen and leads to the more obvious signs of an expanding waistline.

The factors outlined above are major contributors to diabetes and weight management problems. The basic key to this is to really reduce your simple carbs, or instant energy, in favour of more complex carbs (fresh vegetables) and protein (vegetable protein, fish and meats) and remember to create balance with your meals. In taking this approach you will help to boost your glucagon levels to release fat to burn as energy and reduce your insulin exposure as there's not so much blood glucose for the insulin to keep up with.

Avoid Sweeteners - they're not as good as you think they are!

Many dieters turn to sweeteners as an alternative to sugar that helps to cut calorie intake. It's simple to do and there appears to be no downside. However, a US study published in 2008 showed that rats put on weight when they were given food sweetened by artificial sweeteners, unlike their sugar-fed counterparts. The researchers also suggested that this may be a key reason why the obesity epidemic has grown in line with the increased use of artificial sweeteners. Another study, published in 2013, concluded that the artificial sweetener sucralose is able to change the body's response to insulin. It may be that sweeteners react with taste receptors on the tongue that stimulate a reaction in the pancreas and in your gut, which affects your metabolism, even at very low exposure.

It's up to you if you want to include these man-made chemicals in your life, but my advice is to leave well alone. Here's some information on some common sweeteners.

Sorbitol

Sorbitol is about 50 – 70% sweeter than sugar.

This sweetener is often found in chewing gum and some people on weight loss regimes opt to chew gum to keep hunger pains at bay or for 'face entertainment'. It's also found in toothpaste and sweets.

Stomach pains and diarrhoea can be a side effect of high sorbitol consumption. Sorbitol can have a laxative effect because it is not absorbed very well and this means that extra water is brought into the intestine, which will cause diarrhoea. This is not a weight loss strategy as losing a lot of fluid from your body on a consistent basis will ultimately cause dehydration, which can become serious.

Sorbitol comes from a group of sweeteners called sugar alcohols and these include: xylitol and mannitol, which are known to cause bloating, diarrhoea and weight gain.

Saccharin

This sweetener is very low in calories and is about 200-700 times sweeter than sugar.

This is the sweetener that has been around the longest. It has a chequered history as it was linked with causing bladder cancer in rats as far back as the 1970's but this link was marginalised by the Calorie Control Council who said that it could not be justified.

This was the sweetener used in the 2008 study mentioned above and concluded that the animals gained weight.

Aspartame

A low to zero calorie sweetener that is 200 times sweeter than sugar.

This is a sweetener that was discovered by mistake by a scientist who was working to develop a stomach ulcer drug. Aspartame is absorbed by the body, unlike Sorbitol, and aspartame's by-products (how it is broken down by the body) can produce brain damage in the long term. If you have diabetes, smoke or have high blood pressure you may also experience a more pronounced reaction to aspartame. Please don't give this to children.

Side effects can include headaches, seizures,

depression, loss of eyesight and weight gain. It can cause weight gain because it stimulates secretion of insulin, which will drop your blood sugar and have you reaching for some instant energy foods, sabotaging your willpower and dieting aims.

Just in case I leave you with any doubt about aspartame you might want to read Russell Blaylock's book, *Excitotoxins: the taste that kills,* which will give you the low down on aspartame. But in the meantime I'd like to tell you about one of Dr Patrick Kingsley's patients reported in the magazine, *What Doctor's Don't Tell You* (2013).

Henry was 14 and walking on crutches, he had seen four neurologists (brain/nervous system doctors) who had all diagnosed him with the one of the youngest cases of Multiple Sclerosis that had been seen in the UK. Dr Kingsley took a detailed history but nothing of any import seemed to be revealing itself until they decided to take a break whilst Dr Kingsley saw another patient and Henry was to have an intravenous nutrient infusion. As they took the break Henry asked his Mum for a drink. Mum produced a bottle of Diet Coke, reporting to Dr Kingsley how much Henry loved it and that he drank at least two bottles every day. Dr Kingsley had suddenly found the missing piece of his puzzle because he knew that some American children had developed MS-type symptoms when they had consumed a lot of Diet Coke. Henry's Mum reported that he had started to drink it when a vending machine was installed at his school two or three years before and at least two other boys at the school had developed MS like Henry and no one knew why.

Henry stopped drinking the diet drink immediately and went through the unpleasant withdrawal symptoms of headache and low back pain, but after just six months he had recovered completely to be the fit and active 14-year-old that he should be.

Acesulfame K

This sweetener is zero calorie and is 200 times sweeter than sugar.

This is another sweetener that has been linked with cancer in animal studies but on a more immediate note it has also been linked with stimulating insulin secretion and therefore potential weight gain.

Long term exposure to this sweetener may lead to headaches, visual disturbances, depression and nausea to mention a few problems.

This is not a full discussion about sweeteners but I hope these brief bytes of information spell out to you that sweeteners may provide an option to reduce calorie intake but all they do is mess around with your body chemistry, which makes feeling well and energised a much harder thing to achieve and maintain.

The Ovaries

The ovaries are part of the female reproductive system and the hormones from your ovaries: oestrogen, testosterone and progesterone can be linked with hormone-related problems that can be linked to weight management difficulties.

Polycystic Ovaries

This is a very common hormone imbalance that affects many women of reproductive age. The problem can manifest with differing levels of severity but the basic problem areas can be:

Excess testosterone (and sometimes DHEAS, an adrenal hormone with male characteristics) linked with depression, acne and increased facial or body hair;

Excess oestrogen linked with PMS/mood swings, water retention;

Excess oestrogen causing increased insulin secretion, dropping blood sugar and causing sugar cravings;

Excess oestrogen causing increased Thyroid

Binding Globulin (TBG) secretion, making thyroid hormone unavailable and slowing metabolism.

This is a problem that I see quite regularly in my clinic and unfortunately it's very under-diagnosed, but that might be a good thing. The usual medical solutions are the Contraceptive Pill (to suppress ovulation), perhaps an anti-androgen (a male hormone blocker) if the facial/body hair is too much of a problem and a diabetes drug if high levels of insulin are part of the picture. The drugs do not solve the problem - they deal with the symptoms.

There are more natural approaches that can make a profound and lasting difference to women with this problem and looking at diet and lifestyle can be of major assistance in easing the hormonal imbalances mentioned above.

PMS

For a lot of women the time before your period includes the uncomfortable experience of water retention and tender breasts. This is because one of the characteristics of the hormone oestrogen is to retain fluid. It can be upsetting to find that clothes don't fit properly and the scales are giving you a number that is significantly higher than a couple of days before. If you're on a diet your resolve can disappear or at least be severely challenged.

Oestrogen can also impact insulin secretion and this is why many women get the chocolate munchies before their period. This is probably the most common problem for women and it's a combination of factors: excess oestrogen and a deficiency of progesterone due to a lack of ovulation – most likely due to stress.

Most women think that they ovulate every month if they are not on the Pill. This is not the case, there are a number of things that can affect ovulation and a main factor is stress. A high cortisol level will stop you from ovulating and if you don't ovulate you don't get the benefit of the balancing hormone to oestrogen, progesterone. The months when you do ovulate you probably experience a noticeably less problematic period.

Progesterone should not to be confused with the progestins or progestogens found in the Pill. These hormones are synthetic cousins that do not have the same effects as the natural hormone and can even be linked with causing problems such as acne and facial hair because they are chemically quite similar to testosterone, the male hormone.

PMS can cause you to feel moody and sleep can be a problem, which can make matters worse. PMS includes the physical problems of: sugar cravings, water retention, bloating and, potentially a slower metabolism (less calorie burn and less energy). All of these things can impact your resolve and ability to stay on track with your diet.

The Testes

Carrying extra weight for men is a major feminiser - body fat is a harbinger of oestrogen creation. If a man's body has a higher level of oestrogen it will mean that he has less active testosterone and a relative excess of oestrogen to testosterone, which will cool a man's libido, increase risk factors for heart disease as well as increase his likelihood of putting on weight.

Testosterone is the main male hormone that is produced in the testes and it will naturally decline as a man ages but if this is combined with weight gain and resulting higher levels of oestrogen, testosterone's impact can become very muted. Testosterone is an anabolic, or building hormone that will promote the production of bodily protein for the growth of tissues, promoting increased muscle mass and strength, energy and bone density. Maintaining healthy testosterone levels will have positive impacts on:

> Physical and mental energy - better blood sugar regulation;
> Reduced risk of heart disease;
> Less abdominal fat;
> A more lean physique;

all of which are winners when it comes to weight loss and wellbeing.

This is not a comprehensive or formalised run down of what happens hormonally but I hope it's enough to give you a broad understanding as we progress on to discuss some particular areas of hormone influence when it comes to weight management.

WEIGHT LOSS WINNERS

&

DIETING DOWNFALLS

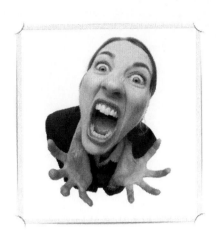

DIETING DOWNFALL – YOUR STRESS

Do these problems apply to you?

Weight gain around the middle	yes/no
Anxiety/nervousness	yes/no
Sugar or salt craving	yes/no
Increased feelings of depression	yes/no
Loss of libido	yes/no
Memory and thinking problems	yes/no
Decreased muscle mass	yes/no
Difficulty sleeping	yes/no
Sugar cravings	yes/no
Fertility problems	yes/no
Blood pressure problems	yes/no
Rapid ageing	yes/no
Dizziness	yes/no

Allergies	yes/no
Fatigue and loss of stamina	yes/no
Aches and pains	yes/no
Low blood sugar	yes/no

If you have answered yes to more than 3 of the above problems you are likely to be suffering from the effects of stress, so let's look at what stress is. (If you have answered yes to questions: fatigue and loss of stamina, allergies, rapid ageing, blood pressure problems, decreased muscle mass, feelings of depression and weight gain around the middle, the effects of stress have been with you for some time.)

Stress - we've all got it, haven't we?

We can be quick to dismiss stress as a foregone conclusion of a busy lifestyle or by comparing it to another person's stress. In both cases it's wrong and perhaps what makes it worse is that conventional medicine has no means of recognising the impact of stress outside the psychological or psychiatric model. The concept of stress as a genuine wellbeing issue and as a precursor to disease still has to work its way into generally accepted clinical practice (certainly in the UK). (NB in July 2013 there were nearly 2,200 published studies on PubMed, the US National Library of Medicine, if the search 'stress and adrenal health' is made.)

Usually, when stress becomes an issue for someone, it's considered to be a mental health problem and the individual may be referred by their family doctor to a Psychologist or a Psychiatrist. I know that many people don't know the difference between a psychologist and a psychiatrist so let's straighten that out.

A psychologist is a non-medically qualified individual, who may or may not have a PhD that entitles them to be addressed as Dr. They deal mainly in talking therapies and looking at behaviours.

A psychiatrist is a medically qualified doctor who has specialised in mental health. They deal mainly in seeing mental health problems as biochemical imbalances in the brain that may be treated with drugs. They may work with talking therapy but may refer to a psychologist for this part of a treatment program.

Understanding Stress

Stress is something that affects us all, all the time, and it's so much better to understand a bit more about it because, when it comes to weight loss, stress can make you eat the wrong foods.

Physical Stress

When you are ill, or have an ongoing hormone

imbalance your physical body is functioning under stress.

When you exercise you are putting your body under stress. We want this to be positive stress but sometimes, if you are asking for more than your body can give, at the gym or on a run, you will be putting your body under negative stress.

Mental and Emotional Stress

Sometimes life is filled with problems, problems, problems and this can create a lot of mental and emotional stress that can turn into distress in areas of life such as:

Finances;
Work;
Relationships;
Bereavement.

Sensitivity and resilience with regard to these problems can depend upon:

hormone balance;
your personal history of life events;
where your personal stress threshold is sitting.

What do I mean by this last point? I have a little analogy that I like to use to described how you may be experiencing stress and it goes like this ...

Response to stress mainly relates to adrenal gland performance, as we discussed earlier, and when your adrenals are in a good place, functioning well with good capacity, it's like you are walking down the motorway of life in the centre lane. The traffic of life is coming towards you, you can see it coming and it doesn't matter if it's a truck, a car or a pedestrian (or, in other words, one of life's big events or a smaller one). You can comfortably take appropriate action, and switch lanes, to avoid being metaphorically flattened.

However, if your adrenals have become worn out and tired over years of constant demands, that big three lane road has narrowed to become a winding country lane with high mud banks. This shift in your situation means that you are no longer able to look ahead and anticipate what's coming at you in life until it's nearly upon you and then it doesn't matter what it is, it knocks you over so that you are constantly picking yourself up and dusting yourself off to start again. This is very tiring and stressful and creates a big sense of vulnerability that explains why very small things can send you into tearfulness, or hysteria or a tearful rage. It's all over-reaction and you know it, but it's all too much to handle. So what's gone wrong?

This is not about your mental health alone – so many people are so relieved to hear that – it's also to do with your adrenal health and capacity. But the trouble is that the unhappiness and guilt of living in this uncomfortable place can drive you to eat (for comfort or solace) or drink to numb the pain. This is a significant example of how your hormones can ambush all your good intentions when you are at your most vulnerable.

DIETING DOWNFALL – *stress makes you crave sugary and salty snacks.*

DIETING DOWNFALL – *stress interferes with thyroid hormone function.*

DIETING DOWNFALL – *stress interferes with sleep and thinking abilities.*

DIETING DOWNFALL – *stress is linked to problems with depression and anxiety.*

DIETING DOWNFALL – *tired adrenals will enhance feelings of vulnerability and helplessness.*

DIETING DOWNFALL – *tired adrenals will see you reaching for energy foods to keep going*

Hormonally speaking what does this all mean?

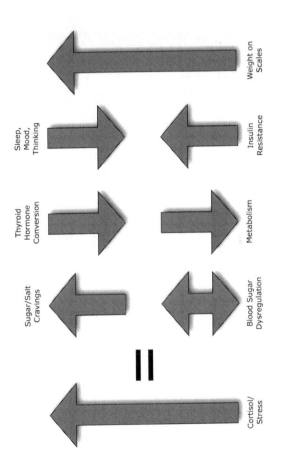

Raised cortisol and stress can really upset the weight management picture, so let's examine the diagram in more depth.

Cortisol will help to provide your body with the energy it's craving by making glucose in the liver from amino acids, which are the building blocks of proteins. This might sound like a good idea when it comes to weight loss as your body appears to be drawing on its own reserves. But let's look further at other knock on relationships ...

The high cortisol will also suppress insulin secretion *and* it causes insulin resistance by blocking insulin from its receptors or docking stations. This means that the energy/blood sugar can't get into your cells and your body thinks that it's starving and sends out messages for you to eat, causing sugar cravings.

An additional factor with higher levels of cortisol is that it will interfere with thyroid hormone conversion and this is something that I discuss in more depth in the chapter on *Metabolism*. Briefly, thyroid hormone (T4) needs to convert to a more powerful cousin (T3) in order to have effective thyroid action around the body. If cortisol is high the conversion process is disrupted and a weaker version of the hormone is created (reverse T3). Having a low level of your most active thyroid hormone can cause you to experience a slower metabolism and therefore gain weight amongst other thyroid related problems such as constipation, depression, anxiety and higher cholesterol levels. Thyroid hormone also needs appropriate levels of cortisol in the blood stream for it to connect with its receptors or docking stations.

Finally, perhaps you can begin to appreciate the mental and emotional impacts of the hormone imbalances discussed above:

If your body thinks it's starving you're going to be irritable;

If your thyroid hormones aren't being effective on a regular or sustained basis, you might feel depressed or anxious;

If your cortisol is high, it's going to affect your thinking and memory as well as sleep. Poor sleep can mean that you start each day feeling fatigued. High cortisol is also linked with depression and anxiety.

All of the above aspects of your hormone health and related to stress can cause some serious dieting downfalls no matter what efforts you're making with calorie counting.

WEIGHT LOSS WINNER - *don't add stress into your life by going on a diet regime that radically changes your eating and shopping habits.*

WEIGHT LOSS WINNER - *try to introduce a way of doing some regular light exercise to disperse physical tension.*

WEIGHT LOSS WINNER - *do a daily life audit to see where your stress points are and see what you can do to change things.*

WEIGHT LOSS WINNER - *reduce stimulants gradually and don't use alcohol to numb feelings of stress.*

WEIGHT LOSS WINNER - *be proactive in managing your meals, reduce addictive carbs.*

Hormonally speaking what does this all mean?

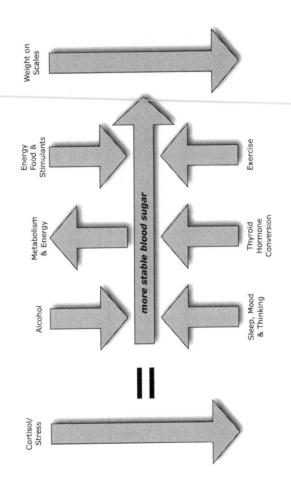

Weight on Scales

Energy Food & Stimulants

Metabolism & Energy

Alcohol

more stable blood sugar

Exercise

Thyroid Hormone Conversion

Sleep, Mood & Thinking

Cortisol/Stress

Going on a new diet brings excitement and anticipation through novelty and hopes of a slimmer, happier you. In reality a different diet that involves a new shopping list, new cooking methods and even new kitchen equipment can be expensive and stressful. Even diets that involve pre-packaged meals can introduce levels of stress because whilst they're easy from the preparation point of view they will often leave you feeling unsatisfied and perhaps uncomfortably out of pocket, which is stressful and adds to the opportunity for hormone hijack. Doing things that reduce stress at this time will contribute significantly to your success in weight loss. Take a look at my *More Tips & Tricks* chapter for ideas about how to reduce the stresses in your life.

An area that many dieters feel pressure is with regard to exercise. Exercise is a tricky thing to manage when it comes to stress and the adrenal glands. I hear from many of my clients how they've been going to the gym in an effort to *find* more energy. They often complain about how hard it is and when we get their adrenal test results back it becomes clear that they were asking their body to do something that it doesn't have the capacity to give.

If you have tired adrenals you may be finding it so difficult to get up in the morning let along drag yourself off to the gym and push yourself into intensity workouts (whether they are strength or cardio). These activities increase the stress your body experiences, pushing up your cravings for sugar and salt and creating profound fatigue that impacts your ability to make good food choices. In order to respect your adrenals and give yourself time for them to recover, exercise needs to be gentle and not overly demanding. Try yoga, swimming (not thrashing up and down doing the crawl!), or walking - try what appeals to you. See my *The Problems with Exercise* chapter for more ideas and tips. The key is always to start with something that you know you can achieve in terms of time and energy output. Don't set yourself up to fail before you begin. As your fitness improves, your ability to handle stress will improve, your energy levels will improve and so will your mood - it's a win-win that will have you smiling.

Stressful responses during your day can also catch you out so initially it's worth spending time each evening reviewing your day and making a few notes. As you look back through your days you may be able to see a pattern emerging that suggests a pressure point or two in your day. which causes you to reach for the wrong food or drink.

Is it when you get home from work that you start to stress about the family chores ahead of you?

Is it that you carry the stresses of the day into your evening allowing your mood and stressed disposition to create tension in relationships at home that cause you to turn to food or alcohol for solace?

Is it lunchtime, after you missed breakfast, that you reach for the crisps and chocolate to restore your energy and mood to get you through the afternoon?

Is it breakfast when all the sugary children's cereals come out of the cupboard to tempt you? (NB - don't give your kids sugar for breakfast, think of their metabolic fire!)

Do you finish your children's uneaten food because you don't want to waste it?

What are your Pressure Points?

The use of stimulants is all around us and the options have grown enormously in the last decade or so:

Coffee shops on every corner;

High caffeine soft drinks;

High sugar "alcopops";

Processed foods and take-aways with high levels of salt, sugar and MSG (monosodium glutamate is a brain stimulant, that can increase your appetite by making you feel hungry sooner);

the list goes on. Look at your food diary and assess where you can easily make improvements by keeping things as simple and basic as possible, don't over-complicate your life. See my *More Tips & Tricks* chapter for suggestions here.

Alcohol can be a prop when you feel that stress is overwhelming you, even a little stress can be too much. We all know that too much alcohol is not good and we've all used alcohol as a way of relaxing, to have 'fun', to numb feelings of stress, upset, anger, anxiety …, but sometimes it becomes a habit. Habits have an unconscious element to them that have you turning to foods and drinks without thinking and it's worth remembering that higher cortisol levels will impair your thinking and memory abilities. If you are truly desperate for an alcoholic drink (a bad sign in itself) try letting a square of chocolate dissolve in your mouth as an alternative to that drink. Granted, it's not a perfect solution but if it helps you curb your appetite for alcohol it's a step in the right direction. This is a tip that is recommended to recovering alcoholics by Alcoholics Anonymous. There are some interesting hypotheses on this but I think that it's a combination of factors including boosting blood sugar, insulin (energy), serotonin (feel better) and oxytocin (have a hug) levels that helps you to 'fill the hole' that alcohol can appear to fill. So make sure that you also sit down with your favourite hot or cold drink so that you also create the 'space' or 'you time' that the alcoholic drink also seems to give you. The urge will pass and then you have a mini-triumph of your own.

Being proactive with your food plans also helps you to manage your appetite and reactive stress from hunger. It also helps you to make better choices. Here are some useful tips:

Make meal menus and keep it simple don't try to create a complicated week for yourself;

Create snack options for the low point in your day - an apple, a few nuts, a protein shake;

Keep your menu to real food, no processed or packet meals;

Try to have set meal times so that you know what you're doing and it will help you to manage your food expectations;

Try not to eat between meals but if you need to manage your low energy dips do it with a pre-emptive healthy snack;

Make it a rule not to eat after a certain time in the evening. This will help your body to rest at night. Going to bed on a stomach that is still working its way through a late night snack or a late evening meal can keep you awake and cause problems with sleep and then fatigue the next day.

Simplifying life on as many levels as you can will really help to reduce the feelings of stress and pressure, support better energy levels and a happier you.

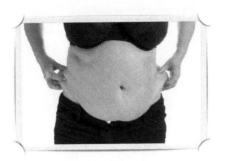

DIETING DOWNFALL – YOUR METABOLISM

Do these problems apply to you?

Sugar or salt craving	yes/no
Cold body temperature	yes/no
Loss of libido	yes/no
Memory and thinking problems	yes/no
Depression and/or anxiety	yes/no
Low blood pressure	yes/no
Dizziness	yes/no
Allergies	yes/no
Fatigue and loss of stamina	yes/no
Aches and pains	yes/no
Low blood sugar	yes/no
Little or no weight loss	yes/no
Constipation	yes/no
Dry skin	yes/no

| Headaches | yes/no |
| Unusual or prolonged fatigue | yes/no |

If you have answered yes to more than 3 of the above problems you are likely to be suffering from a slow metabolism that might be as a result of hormonal imbalance.

Starting at the Beginning - Metabolism and Energy

Metabolism is a term that is used to describe the breaking down of your food and drink (and other things ingested or absorbed by your body) as well as the making of bodily components such as peptides and proteins to maintain and repair your body. This process creates and expends energy at the cellular level. The speed of your metabolism, or metabolic rate, depends on the availability of thyroid hormones, not just the performance of your thyroid gland in pushing out an appropriate level of thyroid hormone, T4 (thyroxine).

Low energy and tiredness go with an inability to lose weight that may be related to a slower metabolism, but you might also be on the Carb Yo-Yo Routine and complementing it with a few alcoholic drinks because you're not sleeping very well. The Carb Yo-Yo Routine messes around with your blood sugar levels sending them up and down as well as helping to lay fat around the middle, changing your shape and raising your risk factors for heart disease and diabetes. If your sleep is disrupted because you're running this boom bust energy machine and using alcohol as a way to relax your body and mind for sleep, you end up suppressing your insulin production and adding more confusion to your metabolic fire. Managing stress and regulating your food intake more effectively are so important to overcoming possible problems with metabolism and energy levels, but you still might be someone with thyroid hormone dysfunction.

I see so many people that complain of weight gain without reason, or report the inability to lose weight on a diet often blaming a slow metabolism. Some clients tell me that their doctor did a thyroid test that came back 'normal', whilst others just put it down to getting older. There are reasons why your thyroid hormone function may be causing a slowed metabolism even though your doctor is unable to identify it. Medicine doesn't have all the answers because it may be more to do with the way in which thyroid hormones are functioning rather than what your doctor is looking for, which is a disease process. However, doctors who rely on TSH (Thyroid Stimulating Hormone) and fT4 (free Thyroxine) testing will not discover a thyroid hormone function problem and may perhaps offer SSRI anti-depressants to help with the feelings of depression and anxiety that can often go with undetected thyroid hormone problems. Unfortunately these drugs are likely to contribute to weight management problems. The key is to address the thyroid hormone situation.

DIETING DOWNFALL – *your stress hormone and energy regulation.*

DIETING DOWNFALL - *factors that can affect thyroid hormone function causing fatigue and lack of weight loss.*

DIETING DOWNFALL – *fatigue is a major reason why people are unable to make better food choices and opt for processed foods.*

DIETING DOWNFALL – *fatigue is a major reason why people cannot find willpower.*

DIETING DOWNFALL – *fatigue is a major reason why people opt out of exercise.*

Hormonally speaking what does this all mean?

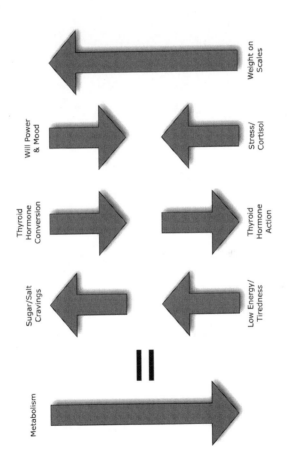

Your metabolism can slow down, which can have effects that draw you deeper into weight gain hell. Problems with thyroid hormone conversion and action as well as stress, or the effects of cortisol, are significant reasons for:

Your metabolism slowing down, making weight loss an up hill battle;

Your energy levels flagging, encouraging you to reach for sugar-based foods;

Your mood to drop and with it your motivation; and,

Your memory and ability to think properly may have you feeling that you can't cope.

Does this picture sound familiar to you? Needless to say they are major downfalls to dieting success.

So what's going on when it comes to thyroid hormone function?

T4 is the main hormone secreted by the thyroid gland and this needs to be converted to T3 to be really useful in sending the thyroid hormone messages to your tissues, including your brain. The trouble is that thyroid hormone action can be interfered with by a number of saboteurs.

Here are the possibilities:

Your T4 is not converting properly to T3

Your main thyroid hormones are T4 (Thyroxine) and T3 (Triiodothyronine) and chemically they are made up of L-Tyrosine (an amino acid) and 4 molecules of iodine, or, L-Tyrosine and 3 molecules of iodine if it's T3. T3 is by far the most active thyroid hormone – low levels will mean that you suffer with underactive thyroid problems without having an underactive thyroid condition.

(Interestingly, even people who have been diagnosed with an underactive thyroid and take synthetic Thyroxine (the usual prescribed replacement hormone) can have this problem, causing continual low thyroid symptoms that necessitate constant blood testing and tweaking of their prescription, often to no avail.)

High levels of cortisol, your stress hormone, will interfere with the conversion of T4 to T3. High cortisol will cause your T4 to convert to rT3 (reverse T3), which is a much weaker and therefore less effective hormone.

Nutritional deficiencies can also affect the ability of your hormones to function properly here.

Stress and the hormone cortisol is impeding the function of your T3

> High or low levels of cortisol in the blood stream caused by either: ongoing stress that is causing your adrenals to secrete a lot of cortisol; or, low levels because your adrenals are now flagging and unable to keep up with demands. Both of these scenarios interfere with thyroid hormone's ability to connect with tissue and it can be an ongoing problem.

Hormone contraceptives lowering availability of your thyroid hormone.

> This is discussed more fully in the next chapter, but higher levels of oestrogen will stimulate secretion of a protein called Thyroid Binding Globulin (TBG), which will bind to thyroid hormone, making it less available for your body to use.

What all this means is that you can be experiencing the effects of an underactive thyroid without having a diseased thyroid gland. I know that many of my clients feel a great sense of relief when they see their test results and have this scenario explained because they were convinced that something was going on with their thyroid but their doctor had insisted that it was normal. Let's look at what can be done to support your metabolism.

WEIGHT LOSS WINNER - *address nutritional deficiencies that affect thyroid hormones.*

WEIGHT LOSS WINNER - *look at your stress factors.*

WEIGHT LOSS WINNER - *look at hormone contraceptive use.*

WEIGHT LOSS WINNER - *support mood and sleep.*

Hormonally speaking what does this all mean?

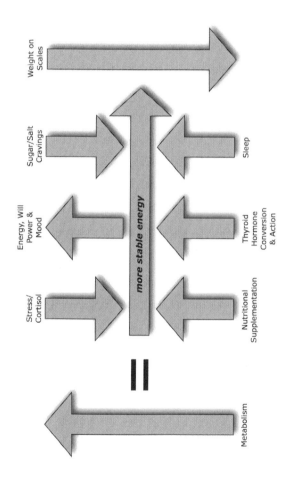

There are some key nutritional deficiencies that can impact your thyroid hormones and these deficiencies aren't necessarily obvious, but they are likely to be quite common. Nutritional deficiencies, particularly zinc and selenium, can mean that your body doesn't have the necessary minerals to convert your T4 to T3.

Zinc is used in many enzymatic processes in the body and is important for:

> Supporting the immune system;
>
> Enhancing the actions of Vitamin D;
>
> Hormones – it's an essential part;
>
> Balancing blood sugar and insulin;
>
> Formation of bone and skin;
>
> Converting thyroid hormone into its more active form (T3);
>
> Promoting thyroid activity.

Things that deplete zinc:

> Caffeinated drinks like tea, coffee, colas, etc;
>
> Steroid-based medication;

Diuretics (if not prescribed for medical reasons they can be a favourite of dieters);

The antibiotic tetracycline (or another group, fluoroquinolones) will interfere with absorption.

Don't take any more than 25mg per day to support your body's needs. The best forms of zinc for absorption are zinc citrate or zinc picolinate.

Selenium is another essential micro-mineral that is important for:

Thyroid function;
Immune system;
Reducing toxicity from heavy metals;
May help to prevent heart disease and cancer.

Don't take selenium with Proton Pump Inhibitors, used to treat reflux, or anti-histamines. Selenium can be toxic at high levels so the usual dosage is 200 mcg per day.

Taking a good quality multi vitamin and mineral formulation can be a good way to provide your body with ongoing nutritional support to your diet.

When it comes to optimal thyroid function stress and cortisol are very important influences. Carefully review the preceding chapter on stress. However, if you are someone who takes Thyroxine be aware that general medical practice doesn't tend to observe the importance of cortisol in thyroid function. It's not uncommon for me to see test results of clients that illustrate how the prescription of thyroid medication has increased the processing of cortisol through the liver, putting more stress on the adrenals to replace it, which can lead to a further lowering of adrenal reserve so that there's not enough cortisol in the blood for thyroid hormone to connect with its receptors. The outcome is that the individual has enough thyroid hormone but the hormone can't connect to tissue in effective amounts. The underactive thyroid symptoms continue, including problems with weight management.

The influence of the Pill and HRT is another area that is not generally recognised with regard to thyroid hormone influence and this is addressed more fully in the next chapter on *Oestrogen*. If you are experiencing problems with weight management it may be because your contraception or HRT has slowed your metabolism and increased your ability to retain fluid.

Supporting your thyroid hormones is a major influence in your metabolism that will enhance many positive areas of your health and wellbeing. This can mean a huge difference in your success - both short and long term - in achieving your weight loss goals.

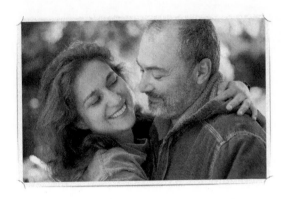

DIETING DOWNFALL – YOUR OESTROGEN

Questionnaire

Do these problems apply to you on a regular basis - for girls?

Mood swings	yes/no
Anxiety/nervousness	yes/no
Depression	yes/no
Water retention	yes/no
Fibroids	yes/no
Lumpy breasts	yes/no
Tender breasts	yes/no
Cold body temperature	yes/no
Sugar cravings	yes/no
Headaches	yes/no
Weight gain at the hips	yes/no

Do these problems apply to you on a regular basis - for guys?

Increased need to pee	yes/no
Decreased libido or sex drive	yes/no
Breast tissue growth	yes/no
Cold body temperature	yes/no
Weight gain at the hips	yes/no
Increased irritability	yes/no
Prostate problems (for older guys)	yes/no

If you have answered yes to more than 3 of the above problems you are likely to be suffering with an oestrogen dominance problem, which may be because of your own hormone imbalance (girls and guys) or it may be because of the Pill or HRT if you are a woman.

What is Oestrogen?

Oestrogen is the general name for a group of hormones that is responsible for promoting the formation of female sexual characteristics (such as breasts) and the regulation the menstrual cycle. There are many other things that oestrogen is involved in but for the purposes of our discussion the above mentions will suffice.

Oestrogen is a general name for three types of oestrogen found in the body: oestrone (east - rone) is the oestrogen produced in fat cells and naturally affects men and women, especially if you are overweight, it's also produced by the ovaries and adrenals; oestradiol (east-ra-dial) is produced by the ovaries and is the dominant hormone found in younger women before the menopause; and, in men it's produced in the testes and the adrenals; oestriol (east-riol) is the oestrogen produced by the placenta during pregnancy - this is the weakest form of oestrogen.

There are also other types of oestrogen that we can be exposed to intentionally or through the environment:

Phytoestrogens are plant oestrogens so-called because they are elements of the plant that have oestrogen-like activity. Phytoestrogens can be found in plants such as: Black Cohosh, Damiana, Flax Seed, Red Clover, Wild Oats, Soy and Sage.

Xenoestrogens, or foreign oestrogens, can be found in a wide variety of pesticides and other chemicals, including cosmetic products.

Synthetic, or man-made oestrogens is another group, which includes the Pill and HRT.

At this point men may be thinking that is chapter doesn't really apply to them but you'd be sadly mistaken. Oestrogen exposure for men is a growing problem and this is illustrated through the statistics for breast reduction surgeries in the UK over the last few years. In 2008 there were 323 surgeries on men, in 2009 this number increased to 581, in 2010 there were 741 and by 2011 numbers rose still further to 790; an increase of 244% over these four years. A man's ability to generate oestrogen around the body is enhanced with the more body fat that he carries and the impact can often be seen through a change in body shape, a feminisation, with weight gain at the hips and breast. The increased level of oestrogen in his body will also have a negative impact on testosterone production, increasing the potential impact of the oestrogen and dampening libido as well as increasing risk of stroke, heart disease and prostate problems. The influence of oestrogen on the prostate is only recently being recognised as the focus was on testosterone previously. In Canada, researchers found a strong correlation between the use of the Pill (and HRT) in the female population and increased incidence of prostate cancer. You might wonder how this is connected, but oestrogen is excreted by women in urine, which gets into the water supply.

So, let's now look on the female side of environmental exposure to oestrogen. Whilst higher levels of oestrogen might be more 'natural' to a woman, they increase the oestrogen burden on the body and the potential risk of oestrogen-related cancers such as breast cancer; as well as problems with heavy periods and the risk of uterine fibroid growth. (Fibroids are very common benign growths found in the uterus or womb.)

For both men and women if you are experiencing oestrogen dominance related problems you should be examining where you might be able to reduce your exposure.

DIETING DOWNFALL – *excess body fat will cause higher levels of oestrogen.*

DIETING DOWNFALL – *oestrogen dominance can increase insulin production.*

DIETING DOWNFALL – *taking the Pill or HRT can slow down your metabolism.*

DIETING DOWNFALL – *oestrogen dominance leads to more water retention, which can dramatically affect the scales in any weight loss regime.*

Hormonally speaking what does this all mean?

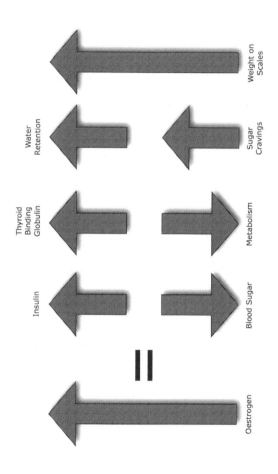

Firstly, whether you are male or female if you are carrying extra weight your body fat will be boosting your oestrogen levels and relatively higher levels of oestrogen will increase secretion of insulin, your blood sugar regulating hormone. Higher levels of insulin mean a drop in blood sugar and when you have a drop in blood sugar, energy levels sink and the body says, give me instant energy now! The quickest form of energy is sugar and the trouble is that sugar will give you the boost but then you fall down the other side of the short-lived boost, which can have you reaching for more instant energy. It's a vicious circle that's not about willpower, it's about your body's calls for energy to think (because the brain needs glucose) and to function and oestrogen levels can play a role.

For women, oestrogen dominance before your period can stimulate chocolate cravings, which may be because of a higher level of insulin dropping blood sugar, but it may also be because oestrogen can affect mood. So the drive can come from a subconscious need to lift your mood with carbs for a boost of serotonin or perhaps your snappy mood has left you feeling guilty and unloveable and you need a hug - some nice sensual eating could give you that boost of oxytocin, your 'hug' hormone.

The same problems can affect women on the Pill and HRT because whilst these drugs suppress ovarian production of oestrogen, the replacement synthetic version is often supplemented to higher than natural levels, causing permanent exposure to higher oestrogen levels, but these are not the only impacts of these drugs on your hormone levels and your weight management issues ...

Higher oestrogen levels, whether caused by the Pill or by your body, will also cause the secretion of higher levels of a protein called Thyroid Binding Globulin (TBG). TBG binds to thyroid hormone making it less available for the body to use. This, in effect, means that you can potentially become a little hypothyroid, slowing down metabolism, creating tiredness, constipation and perhaps feelings of depression.

Look at methods of contraception (or HRT) as not only do higher levels of oestrogen from the Pill contribute to higher levels of TBG, they also stimulate a protein called Sex Hormone Globulin (SHBG), which binds to the sex hormone testosterone to make it less available to the body. This is a significant contributor to a loss of libido, which can come between you and your partner, cause problems between you, leaving you to seek solace in food.

Another major characteristic of the hormone oestrogen is that it encourages fluid retention, which is why you may experience tender breasts, a swollen belly and even headaches. However, generally your body's ability to retain fluid can depend on how hydrated you are as well as what your oestrogen levels are. Fluid retention could cause a difference of perhaps 7lbs in your weight on the scales.

There are also things in your diet and lifestyle that will increase your exposure to oestrogen:

Alcohol consumption – if you are drinking every evening to wind down after a stressful day you are boosting oestrogen levels, in fact, it can temporarily triple oestrogen levels. Alcohol consumption may be a bigger problem than many men and women are prepared to admit. New research (2013) from the University of Sunderland (UK) estimates that 60% of women in more affluent areas of the UK are consuming more than the recommended three units of alcohol per day. It's become a form of reward for doing family chores after work and to relieve stress according to this research, which probably rings true for many people.

Grapefruit diets and grapefruit juice consumption can increase oestrogen levels. If you are on the Pill or HRT this can have a significant impact on your oestrogen levels and increase your risk of developing a blood clot. Grapefruit interferes with your body's ability to break down oestrogen-related drugs such as the Pill and HRT.

Some medications can also increase oestrogen levels, including: pain relievers such as ibuprofen, acetaminophen, aspirin, antibiotics, statins, some commonly prescribed anti-depressants, some blood pressure medications and calcium channel blockers.

NB If you are on a regular prescription for any of these drugs and have concerns about heavy periods or fibroids or other oestrogen-related problems such as endometriosis, fibrocystic breast disease or even breast cancer talk to your doctor about alternatives. Do not simply take yourself off your medication.

Now that we've identified some dieting downfalls of oestrogen let's look at what you can do to achieve some weight loss winners.

WEIGHT LOSS WINNER - *improve the processing of oestrogen through your system.*

WEIGHT LOSS WINNER - *weigh yourself daily, keep a record and note if you feel you are retaining water so that you don't become disheartened.*

WEIGHT LOSS WINNER - *reducing the stress in your life will also help to stabilise blood sugar and, if you're a woman, support ovulation.*

WEIGHT LOSS WINNER - *discuss the dose of your Pill or HRT with your doctor to see if it can be reduced or if there is an alternative.*

Hormonally speaking what does this all mean?

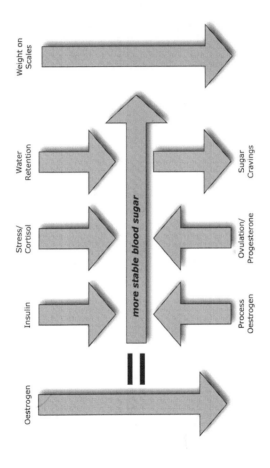

Dietary supplements may help your body to process oestrogen more effectively and this will reduce your overall exposure. Dietary indoles such as DIM (Diindolylmethane) and I3C (Indole-3-carbinole) help to shift the oestrogen balance in favour of 2-hydroxyestrone, a protective and softer oestrogen metabolite (breakdown product), which may support the wellbeing of oestrogen-sensitive tissues.

Dietary indoles are active plant nutrients found in broccoli, cabbage, kale, cauliflower, turnips and brussel sprouts so there's an important reason to eat up your greens, but if you want to go down the supplement route the recommended dosage is 300-800 mg per day. Side effects may be noticed by a few people with problems such as flatulence and nausea, however, a lower dose can help to resolve this. (Antacids and H2 Blockers (such as Zantac) can inhibit the effectiveness of I3C.)

Another supplement that can support the processing of oestrogen is Calcium d-Glucarate, which is a supplemental form of d-Glucaric acid, a natural substance found in many fruits and vegetables such as brussel sprouts, apples, broccoli, cabbage and bean sprouts. Calcium d-Glucarate can help to support the natural excretion of steroid hormones, such as oestrogen, and carcinogens (cancer causing agents) by Phase II liver pathways, which can have a protective role for the immune system. If you want to supplement the recommended dosage is 500-1000 mg per day.

(People on statin medication should be aware that animal studies have shown that d-Glucaric acid can lower cholesterol by as much as 12-15%.)

Dietary indoles and Calcium d-Glucarate can be used by men and women alike.

One benefit of reducing your exposure to oestrogen is that it will help to reduce fluid retention, although there are other reasons that you may be retaining fluid so you may want to get this checked out by your doctor if it is a permanent problem for you. However, by reducing your oestrogen burden you will find that fluid retention related to this will disappear or become very minimal, reducing the weight gain on the scales and the feelings of tightness in your clothes.

Apart from improving your body's ability to process oestrogen it's important to review the impact of stress and the hormone cortisol. Lower stress will help to stabilise your blood sugar, which will help you to stay on track with your good dietary intentions. Also, for girls who menstruate naturally, less cortisol means a higher likelihood of ovulation. Ovulation is not a process that occurs every month as a matter of course, it's dramatically influenced by hormone imbalance and excess cortisol, or stress, will often prevent ovulation. Ovulation brings the balancing effects of the hormone progesterone, which helps to offset the effects of oestrogen and complete the menstrual cycle properly with less problems that relate to PMS.

If this scenario seems familiar to you and you are on the Pill or HRT then should should be talking to your doctor about reducing your dose or coming off it. There are other methods of contraception that offer lower exposure to oestrogen, however, don't swap to progestin-based pills or alternatives as they are a step backwards. (Progestins, or synthetic progesterones, are, as a class of hormonal drug, registered carcinogens – cancer causing agents. It was the Women's Health Trials in the early 2000's in which the progestin arm (or combined oestrogen and progestin HRT) of the trial had to be stopped because of the higher incidence of breast cancer. Remember that the Pill is essentially the same drug combination as HRT. Talk to your doctor about alternatives that might work for you. Try to be non-hormonal and if you are not in a long term relationship go for barrier methods to avoid sexually transmitted infections.

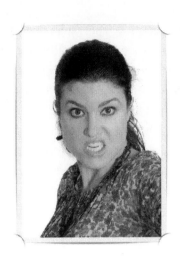

DIETING DOWNFALL – YOUR MOOD

Questionnaire

*Do these problems apply to you on a
regular basis?*

Bouts of depression	yes/no
Feelings of anxiety and/or nervousness	yes/no
Mood swings	yes/no
Irritability	yes/no
Tearfulness	yes/no
Feeling on the defensive	yes/no
Burned out feeling	yes/no
Apathy	yes/no
Overwhelmed/tired	yes/no

If you have answered yes to more than 3 of the above problems you are likely to be suffering with a mood problem that may be cyclical or it may be bothering you on a more permanent basis.

Mood is a major factor in how you feel about looking after yourself on a minute by minute basis and reflects in the choices you make in your diet and lifestyle. It's often the reason why diets can be broken in the blink of an eye. As your mood goes down, your sense of self goes with it, you begin to fall into the 'poor me' trap and the self-talk starts with why you *can* have that piece of cake or the extra helping. You start to justify and organise your thoughts and feelings in order to arrive at the 'right' answer, except that it's often the wrong answer. Frustration and regret settle in too late.

On calorie restriction regimes it's easier to get irritable with others and yourself because you're sending your blood sugar well down when it's been kept high, or yo-yoing, for a long time and irritability is a known relationship to low blood sugar. This is also the time when you can start to feel sorry for yourself or angry, pushing up stress levels, making your body shout even more for some 'feel good' relief. A major influence on your body's feel good factor is food. Food can deliver energy and the carbs that can support your gut's ability to make serotonin (your 'happy' hormone) and the physical sensations of eating can give you the boost of oxytocin that makes you feel hugged, loved and connected again.

We're not going to look at the wider influences of hormone imbalances themselves in this chapter because they are covered elsewhere. What we are going to look at is the Three E's, Emotional Eating, Energy Eating and Entertainment Eating, which illustrate the close connections between how you feel and eating. Understanding this will help you to identify influences and behaviour that can undermine your weight loss aims.

DIETING DOWNFALL – *your mood will predict your vulnerability with regard to the Three E's - which can relate to seeking a boost of: serotonin, oxytocin and/or blood sugar.*

What's Eating You?

Common weight loss hurdles include what I call the Three E's, which are great examples of the hormone influence on weight loss success or failure based on how you feel.

Emotional Eating

Emotional set backs and problems can trigger an eating response that feels hard or impossible to control. These feelings can be heightened by your past experiences making you feel vulnerable and reminding you of a time in your life that you have tried to forget. So you eat or drink to feel comforted.

Sometimes the comforting behaviour is about the fact that something has gone wrong and you feel:

    guilty;
    responsible;
    powerless.

Sometimes it's because someone has hurt you and you feel:

    upset;
    ashamed;
    depressed;
    unloved.

Sometimes it's because you've had a very stressful, busy day where you've been:

    watching the clock;
    trying to make a deadline;
    too much work and too little time.

These are all external events that can and will ramp up your stress hormone (cortisol) levels and if you use food for comfort you will be turning to carbs to:

    Raise your blood sugar (excess cortisol from stress will tell your body you're starving);

Raise your serotonin level (your 'feel good' hormone, which is made when you eat carbs);

To have something nice because you deserve it and need a 'food hug', which will raise your oxytocin level (your 'hug' hormone).

What are your Emotional Eating weaknesses?

Energy Eating

This E attacks when you're tired, stressed or bored and it's a fairly straightforward situation that feels like you *need* something quick to keep you going. This is the time when you might find yourself roaming around the kitchen looking for that quick hit, or decide to go to the vending machine at work or nip out to the corner shop to pick up the packet of instant energy.

Energy dips can happen because you're using too many carbs in your diet, which will give you energy peaks followed by troughs or dips. This behaviour has you reaching for another 'hit' because you're experiencing a low energy period.

Depending on the time of day or what your particular need is, you might look for:

coffee and a pastry (caffeine stimulant and sugar for energy);

soft drink and a bar of chocolate (again this can be a caffeine stimulant and sugar for energy);

soft drink and a packet of crisps (you look for a salty snack if your adrenals are particularly tired, but you've also got the carbs with the crisps and perhaps the caffeine in the soft drink);

tea and cake or a biscuit or three (tea also has caffeine that can give you a boost and plenty of sugar and even fat in the cake or biscuit)!

What are your energy food weaknesses?

Entertainment Eating

Face entertainment with your favourite foods is like a forbidden sensual pleasure - texture, taste and smell. But probably the biggest hit comes from the texture, the feeling of eating. Does it satisfy your mouth-craving to crunch, to wallow in the creaminess, or, to have something chewy; something salty or something sweet?

Eating is a sensual delight that you might be forgetting

to enjoy because you eat in front of the tv, reading, or using your computer or phone, but there's more to eating than you might at first realise. The act of eating and experiencing your food acts as a physical stroking of the body, just like someone touching you, hugging you or even massaging you. The digestive system from mouth to bowel is made from the same germ cells as the skin so the sense of touch is also an important part of your eating experiencing. This action has an important hormonal message because the hormone oxytocin is secreted through touch stimulus and it's your 'hug' or bonding hormone. Oxytocin has been found to be released in both men and women, to similar levels, in response to pleasant warmth and rhythmic touch and helps you to feel calm and relaxed, the opposite of adrenaline and noradrenaline, your fight or flight hormones.

What are your guilty pleasures?

Don't underestimate the power of the Three E's to undermine your motivation and dedication to your dieting and healthy eating intentions.

Hormonally speaking what does this all mean?

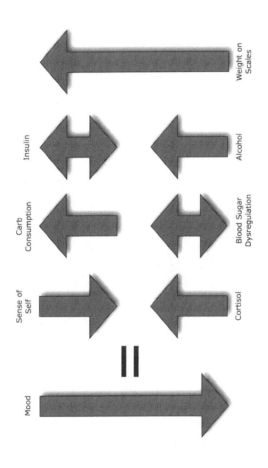

There really is a lot to think about here but when you understand things a bit better you can learn how to take proactive steps or even just knowing what it is helps you to avoid being beaten by it.

The diagram above concentrates on some of the direct influences on your desire to eat:

Low blood sugar can affect you at points during your day, for some it's mid-morning but for many it's that mid to late afternoon slump that hits you hard, leaving you feeling like you want to crawl to a quiet corner and have a sleep. The slump makes you feel tired and irritable but it's the irritability that will often push you to make poor choices about food.

Are you someone who reaches for the glass of wine or beer when you get home from work? If you add alcohol to your mix of low mood, in an attempt to numb the mood or to cheer yourself up, you're heading for a bigger downer not least because alcohol is a depressant but also because it will raise your insulin level, lowering blood sugar even further and this will have you craving carbs! (Just think of all those queues outside fish and chip bars and kebab shops after the night clubs close - they are suffering the effects of raised insulin and low blood sugar!)

These are two examples that help to explain the

hormonal mechanics but when it comes to mood what you're really looking for is to emotionally feel better and this is where the food connections to serotonin and oxytocin come in.

Serotonin

If you have blamed yourself for a binge on chocolate or cake or crisps, well, carbs, then don't be too hard on yourself. Your mood is not something you can ignore or see in isolation. You see your body will drive you to give it what it needs and wants. If your mood is low, your body may have learnt through past experience that eating carbs will give it the right ingredients to make serotonin. A boost in serotonin makes you feel better and can lift your mood.

Not everyone eats when they feel down, it's all part of what you learn about combined with the effects of what you eat and drink. A type of antidepressant medication called Selective Serotonin Re-Uptake Inhibitors prevents your brain using up too much serotonin and feeding on carbs will top up your serotonin in a natural, but not healthy way. On a weight loss regime topping up on carbs can be a really big downfall for some people and it's certainly not a solution for depression, but then neither are SSRI's, which have a listed side effect of weight gain.

Warning: do not suddenly stop antidepressant medication. You do not want or need to be plunged into depths or to suffer considerable withdrawal symptoms. Consult your doctor about a program to come off your medication.

Not all feelings of depression or anxiety can be medicated away and for some counselling is both important and appropriate. If you have something you feel you need to talk about with a suitably qualified professional then trust yourself. I always counsel my clients that they should never judge the magnitude of their inner struggles against those of another as to whether they matter, or are important enough. If they are important, distracting, disturbing, or upsetting enough to you that's all you need to know. Find a professional to talk to.

Oxytocin

Mood can be reflective of a feeling of loneliness or isolation, which leaves you needing a hug or a gentle touch when there's no one around to fulfil that need in the appropriate way. Food can be experienced as a physical stroking of your body as you experience the right textures and sensations in your mouth and then that comforting feeling of the full stomach and subconsciously as it makes its way through your gut. This touch stimulus will stimulate the secretion of oxytocin, which establishes a different level of connection with your food that can become addictive in itself.

A study published in 2012 has advanced knowledge about oxytocin's relationship to weight loss and it found that this hormone has anti-obesity effects, which makes sense if you think about how you feel when you fall in love. Your energy levels go up, your mood improves and hunger subsides as you feed on the food of love!

If you are eating to fill a void of feeling unloved, lonely or isolated this is something that you need to acknowledge and do something about. Think about getting a massage on a regular basis as this can help you to feel more relaxed and enjoy someone's touch to help you overcome feelings of neglect because that's what they are.

All of the above mental/emotional health (mood) problems may be more to do with hormone imbalance than mental instability requiring psychiatric medicines that alter brain chemistry. I know in my clinic many women, in particular, are so relieved when their hormone evaluation comes back and they begin to understand why they feel so bad mentally and emotionally. It is sometimes tragic. I've worked with one woman who used her report to prevent her own 'Sectioning' (enforced admittance) to a psychiatric ward and another woman who, on her recovery, asked her psychiatrist why hormone imbalance was never considered a possibility.

Here are some other hormone explanations for mood problems:

Thyroid hormone deficiency or poor function can be related to depression and anxiety;

Oestrogen dominance can be related to mood swings, irritability, blood sugar lows, depression and anxiety; and,

Stress – this is deemed to be a psychiatric area of medicine (mental health) but recognised effects of high cortisol are anxiety and depression. Anxiety can also be whipped up into full blown panic attacks that can be very uncomfortable. There are psychiatric studies that show that a simple cup of tea or coffee can even induce a panic attack.

Hormone imbalances such as those mentioned above are real and can really impact your mood and general sense of wellbeing yet they are generally not treated effectively and can often be made worse by female hormonal interventions such as the Pill or HRT, or by trying to treat them through mental health routes.

WEIGHT LOSS WINNER - *identify the weak point of your day and do something to change your routine.*

WEIGHT LOSS WINNER - *increase your protein intake.*

WEIGHT LOSS WINNER - *if you feel you need to - talk to someone.*

WEIGHT LOSS WINNER - *identify if you may be under the influence of hormone imbalance.*

Hormonally speaking what does this all mean?

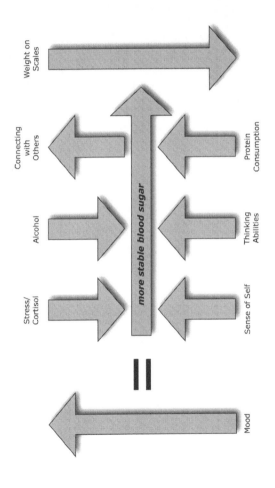

Emotional eating is often a learned behaviour, in other words you did it once and it made you feel better on some level – lesson learnt!

The first thing to do is to identify the weak point of your day.

For example –

1. Is it mornings after everyone has left the house, if you are a stay-at-home Mum?

2. Is it evenings when you sit down in front of the tv?

Or,

3. Is it even just a weekend thing if you live alone?

Once you establish when you are at a vulnerable time then it's time to work out a behaviour changing approach. For example –

If you are Example 1, make sure you distract yourself. Go and get straight into the shower and get dressed up so that you feel more together and in control of your day.

If you are more like Example 2, you could prepare healthy alternatives to the crisps or biscuits, like carrot sticks and hummus. But it can also be about getting out of the mindset of eating whilst watching tv. Does your mouth really need entertaining at the same time as your mind?

Another point worth remembering is that eating a meal or snack in front of the tv will mean that you are not paying attention to the food, you will eat more and probably go back to the kitchen for more because you haven't nourished your body and mind with the sights and smells that contribute to your food enjoyment.

As an Example 3 person, this really means that your feelings of loneliness should be addressed. Look at your local leisure centre and see what classes might be available for you to go out, meet people and get involved. You do not need to bury your feelings under a mound of carbohydrates. Exercise is a good way of naturally boosting endorphins, your very own wellbeing hormones!

Another tip that can help you to be a bit more proactive on the mood front is to give yourself a natural no/low calorie lift with 5-HTP. If used properly and consistently it can boost your serotonin levels to help you feel that you are coping better. See more about this supplement in my *More Tips & Tricks* chapter.

With regard to keeping energy levels more stable include protein in your meal, not only is it slow release energy but it will help to cut insulin levels, to help you to avoid the blood sugar lows that will compromise your mood and ability to make good dietary choices.

I've worked with many women in particular who have lost relationships because of their problems with mood. This is an area that medicine is slow to acknowledge because mood is medicated with drugs and you may be referred to a psychologist for counselling or even a psychiatrist. If you feel that counselling is something you should seek then you are probably right and you should find a suitably qualified professional who is easy to talk to - don't persevere with someone you don't get on with. But, talking to your nearest and dearest is also important as it helps you to feel less isolated and alone. You don't need to bare your soul if that's too much but even sharing your feelings is an important step and if you feel that family is too close then a good friend can be a great boost to keeping you feeling connected, understood and cared about.

Hormone imbalances can be the source of mood problems if they are a regular or consistent part of your life. Different hormone influences can be indicative of different mood states as follows:

Low mood can be a feature of a thyroid problem that is not necessarily the gland failing, it could be poor thyroid hormone function as discussed in other chapters through this book.

Feelings of anxiety and panic attacks can be related to high cortisol levels. These feelings can also be made worse by stimulants such as coffee, cola and tea.

Mood swings can be difficult to pin down but if they catch you off guard when you're feeling stressed out it may related to adrenal fatigue and feelings of vulnerability, provoking an overly defensive-aggressive response. But if you're a girl and notice that mood swings are before your period, it's more likely to be oestrogen dominance.

(This is not an exhaustive list but it will give you an idea of how much your hormones can affect your emotional state and as these areas are discussed more fully elsewhere in the book you can see how things are interconnected.)

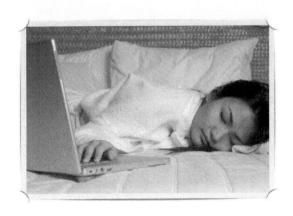

DIETING DOWNFALL – YOUR SLEEP

Questionnaire

Do these problems apply to you on a regular basis?

Disturbed or disrupted sleep	yes/no
Difficulty getting to sleep	yes/no
Take sleeping pills	yes/no
Use alcohol to relax	yes/no
Use caffeine to wake up	yes/no
Have memory problems	yes/no
Foggy thinking	yes/no
Sugar cravings	yes/no

If you have answered yes to more than 3 of the above problems you are likely to be suffering with a sleep problem that is not only keeping you tired and irritable it is increasing your risk of heart disease, diabetes, as well as cancer and creating problems with depression or anxiety. One study has shown that people who have long-term sleep problems have a three times greater risk of dying from any cause. It's important to take your sleep seriously.

Sleep problems are everywhere in our 24/7 environment. It's something you're supposed to do every day of your life but where does it fit in? The world is filled with workers on variable and lengthy shift patterns, tv is available twenty four hours a day, work hours stretch out into your evening and can start as soon as you get up in the morning with mobile devices delivering demanding emails and text messages; let alone having a social life and being part of your family and its needs. Stress and the inability to 'switch off' are common problems.

More and more people are resorting to sleeping pills and in 2011 NHS doctors in the UK handed out 15.3 million prescriptions, but sleeping pills are not a solution to sleep problems and will pose other risks and compromises to your health and wellbeing. Side effects such as: change to your appetite, headaches, constipation, drowsiness, dizziness, confusion and forgetfulness are only a part of the large array of symptoms from these drugs. Withdrawal is another story as it can be extremely difficult to get yourself off these drugs once you start, not just because of chemical addiction but also because of the fear of not sleeping and wondering if you can trust your body again.

Problems with sleep can be a major factor that gets in the way of a successful diet not only because it interferes with your mental faculties (causing forgetfulness and poor decision-making) but also because it will dramatically affect your energy and mood.

Which one are you?

Can't Sleep/Won't Sleep

Going to bed to sleep might be a bit of a battleground for you. As you turn off your light and place your head on your pillow does your mind start chattering away? It's all about yesterday, tomorrow, she said that ..., why did I do that..., oh damn, I forgot so and so ... and so it goes on ... and on. The mind races away on all its little thought loops keeping you from feeling relaxed enough to sleep. Sleep is but a distant dream as the raised cortisol that is keeping your mind active is also suppressing the secretion of your sleep hormone, melatonin.

Sleep can be elusive until finally things quieten down and you can nod off.

Fitful, Light & Disrupted

It might be easy for you to fall asleep when you fall into bed but within an hour or two you wake for the first of many times through the night. It may be that your sleep in between is very light and each time you wake up you're wide awake and the mind is already thinking about the day ahead, things that have annoyed you or distressed you or any number of things that your mind happens to come across.

Quality, deep and restful sleep is a dim and distant memory.

This problem is again linked to cortisol levels playing with your mind and your melatonin levels but what might also be featuring is a disruption of your sleep/wake cycle. This means that your biological pattern (related to your daily and nightly cortisol levels) has become disrupted, probably through poor sleep habits (for example, falling asleep too many times in front of the tv and then expecting to sleep soundly all night). The body learns new behaviour in the end. Your cortisol levels may be staying too high during night time hours for your mind to switch off properly and for your melatonin to be secreted enough to take you off to dreamland.

This cannot be rectified with the use of addictive benzo-based sleeping tablets - drugs.

DIETING DOWNFALL – *raised night time cortisol will keep your mind active preventing the secretion of melatonin, your sleep hormone.*

DIETING DOWNFALL – *lack of quality sleep at night will cause you to reach for quick energy and stimulants to keep you going during the day.*

DIETING DOWNFALL – *difficulty going to sleep can cause you to reach for alcohol as a relaxant.*

DIETING DOWNFALL – *difficulty sleeping will have a marked impact on your mood.*

DIETING DOWNFALL – *difficulty sleeping can increase or even cause problems with foggy thinking and memory.*

Hormonally speaking what does this all mean?

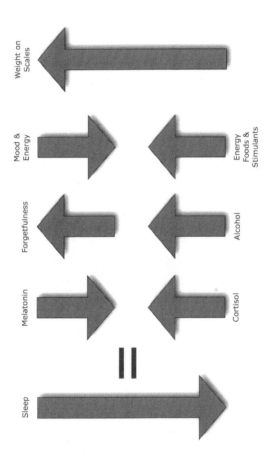

When poor sleep is a constant problem it's very stressful, placing big demands on those poor adrenals again. If lack of sleep is a constant issue it can contribute significantly to the adrenals becoming tired and unable to respond at healthy levels. Tired adrenals contribute to that feeling of getting through each day as though your knuckles are dragging along the floor and that constant feeling of needing to eat to give yourself energy. Quality sleep is essential to your physical, mental and emotional wellbeing.

What do you do when you wake up feeling unrefreshed and hard pushed to get into the day? Many people reach for the caffeine in the form of tea and coffee, perhaps with some sugar (cereal or toast and jam or perhaps a pastry or a croissant or even a breakfast bar if you slept through the snooze alarm). This is how you might be self-medicating your way into the day with caffeine and high octane fuel. The trouble is that these high octane fuels burn quickly and can leave you feeling more tired than when you started, then your body is screaming even harder for more stimulus and more instant energy. Have you read this somewhere before?

This boom during the day might end with a bust at night. When you get home from work you probably experience that 'tired but wired' feeling and you need help climbing down from your caffeine and sugar induced buzz. Perhaps a glass of wine or beer is your wind down after a hard day at work? If this is a reasonable picture of you, you are self-medicating your way down to a more relaxed state of being. It just might be another dieting downfall that is interfering with your sleep.

Following your meal do you fall asleep in the chair with the tv blaring away to itself or your partner? You wake up feeling exhausted and cursing the waste of another evening when you planned to do the ironing and organise yourself for the next day so that, for once, you could feel that you were starting the next day a little ahead. Now, it's all you can do to get a glass of water to quench your dreadful thirst and dry mouth and stumble up the stairs to fall into bed. These evening naps will really disrupt your natural sleep pattern and may be contributing to your wakefulness at night.

WEIGHT LOSS WINNER - *sleep in complete darkness as this will support melatonin secretion.*

WEIGHT LOSS WINNER - *keep regular hours, even at weekends, as much as possible.*

WEIGHT LOSS WINNER - *make it a rule not to eat within two hours of bed time to avoid blood sugar highs that may keep you awake.*

WEIGHT LOSS WINNER - *listen to relaxing music to help you unwind, or, have a hot bath.*

WEIGHT LOSS WINNER - *avoid alcohol and caffeine in the evenings.*

Hormonally speaking what does this all mean?

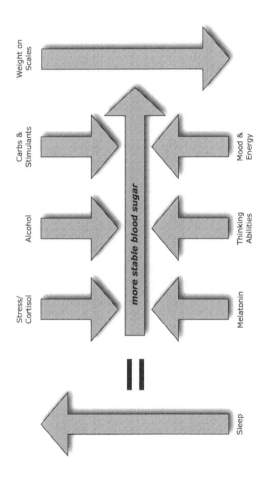

Weight on Scales

Carbs & Stimulants

Mood & Energy

Alcohol

Thinking Abilities

Stress/ Cortisol

Melatonin

more stable blood sugar

=

Sleep

You can make a significant difference to your ability to sleep by using some simple guidelines as follows:

It's important to sleep in complete darkness because this will boost your melatonin secretion, which will help you go into a deeper, more restful sleep. Use black out curtains if you need to block out street lights or invest in an eye mask.

Your ability to go to sleep is also affected by your body's clock and if you continually change your sleep wake hours and take naps it can interfere with a normal pattern. Keep to more regular hours for sleeping and waking so that you support your body's natural rhythms. This is important because your cortisol levels should reflect where you are in your sleep/wake pattern and if your cortisol levels are too high when you go to bed your mind will keep chattering and this is something that causes problems for many people trying to get off to sleep.

If you're having real problems with sleep and feelings of anxiety or tension you might want to look at using a supplement called 5-HTP (L-5-hydroxytryptophan) and you can read more about this in the *More Tips and Tricks* chapter. You may need to experiment to find out what works for you so start small and use it to re-educate your sleep pattern. Start with 50mg dose about half an hour before bed and see if your sleep improves enough. If it's not enough go up to 100 mg but 150mg should be the maximum to help you with sleep. Take it consistently for a month or so before you start to reduce the dose and see how you respond. It should work right from the outset with regard to improving your sleep quality and works by increasing serotonin, which converts to melatonin at night. If you are still having problems at the maximum dose you will need to introduce 5-HTP earlier in the day because you may be carrying intense feelings of stress or anxiety into your evening that cannot be addressed by a late dose of 5-HTP.

NB 5-HTP should not be taken with anti-depressants, weight control drugs or other serotonin modifying drugs or substances known to cause liver damage. People with compromised liver function may not be able to regulate 5-HTP properly.

A good way of supporting relaxation at bed time is an Epsom Salt bath. Epsom Salts or Magnesium Sulphate is not the same thing as salt! The health benefits of Epsom Salts have been known for hundreds of years and the benefit of the mineral is easily absorbed through the skin in a warm, relaxing bath. The magnesium in the salt is known to help to reduce inflammation, relax muscles and tendons and it can help to boost serotonin levels. The sulphate can also help to flush toxins, another benefit when you're on a healthful weight loss regime. Don't use these salts any more than three times per week as they can be quite drying on the skin. If you have a bit of dry skin use a little extra virgin olive oil or coconut oil after your bath as a natural moisturiser. A warm, relaxing bath can help you to quieten the mind and lower your cortisol levels before you go to bed.

Relaxation can also be supported by listening to gentle music at any time of the day, but sounds of nature or the sea or even white noise can also be helpful in helping you to switch off at bed time. The important thing is to establish a good night time routine that helps you to slow things down from the day's hustle and bustle and make the transition between your daytime activities and your night time rest.

Another factor that can be troublesome at bed time is high blood sugar and a good way to avoid it is to resolve not to eat within two hours of going to bed. It can be a good ground rule to instigate as it draws a line under your eating activities for the day and encourages you to take a natural, overnight fast. Foods that boost your sugar levels are important to avoid before bed and, at the other end of the scale, if you try to use alcohol to relax you will cause a drop in blood sugar causing hunger that might keep you awake.

If you find you get hungry at night you need to look at what you're eating in the evening, if it's too high in simple carbs your body is burning your fuel too quickly. Think about your metabolic fire and see what changes you might need to make. You might even like to try making sure that you include some dietary intake of the amino acid L-Tryptophan with the following foods:

pork, cottage cheese, duck, wheat germ or avocado for example. L-Tryptophan is the amino acid that is a building block of serotonin and melatonin.

Giving your body a prod with stimulants to keep it going during the day and then coshing it at night with alcohol is a very unkind way of treating yourself. Be more gentle with yourself during your days and nights could be flowing more easily.

THE PROBLEMS WITH EXERCISE

Exercise can be an elusive and difficult to fit in element of having a healthy lifestyle, but in the words of Edward Stanley, the 15th Earl of Derby (1826 -93).

"Those who think they have not time for bodily exercise will sooner or later have to find time for illness."

What Holds You Back from Taking Your Daily Constitutional?

Taking a walk used to be part of everyone's day as an activity that was good for your body and mind. In fact, nothing has changed - a new study (2013) concluded that people who walk to work have a 40% less risk of succumbing to diabetes when compared with people who drive to work. This information is worth taking on board because it's clear that the UK's problem with diabetes is growing. In 2005/2006 there were 27.1 million prescriptions issued for diabetes (per item), costing the NHS nearly £514 million, by 2012/2013 the number of prescription items has gone up to 42.5 million with a cost of just over £764 million. These escalating costs for a lifestyle-related disease are costing the nation dearly as well as the individual. Did you know that the most common reason for an amputation surgery is not accidental injury but diabetes?

So, apart from a general reluctance there might be a number of genuine reasons why fitting exercise into your routine might be a challenge.

Your thyroid hormones are not functioning optimally, which compromises mood, motivation, energy and stamina;

Your adrenals are quite tired or stressed, which interferes with energy levels as well as the ability to handle stress. (With this problem you could be wearing yourself out each day with the bodily tension you're hanging on to.);

Lack of sleep means that you're too tired to get through the day let alone do exercise as well.

There are also excuses that don't make the grade; for example,

Not enough time to fit it in;
Too many other commitments;
No spare cash to pay for a class or membership.

The most important thing to do is to work out what sort of exercise motivates you and, to start with, what you can incorporate into your day. You can go from there.

If you have real hormone deficiencies that are causing problems with your wellbeing then you need to address them, but you can still do some gentle exercise.

The following are easy, cheap and convenient exercise regimes to start you on your way;

1. 5 minutes out from your front door and 5 minutes back:

at the beginning of the day can serve to get you revved up and oxygenated for the day ahead;

at the end of the day (before you take a coat or jacket off when you come home from work) can help you to make a better transition from work to home life and allow you to breath, release bodily tension and clear your mind (instead of that calorific wine or beer).

2. Get a yoga/tai chi/exercise/dance DVD that you can use at home. Start by scheduling 2 evenings or mornings a week combined with 1 above.

3. March in front of the tv when the adverts come on during your tv program. Do that for 2 or 3 ads and you may have done 6 – 10 minutes exercise without thinking about it. All you have to do is stand up.

4. Use stairs and walk wherever you can instead of lifts or cars or buses.

5. In the supermarket car park, park as far away as you can from the door. A walk to the door will allow you to set your mind about your intentions when you get there. It will also increase your movement total for the day.

6. Use your house stairs as your very own 'Stairmaster' – plan to go up and down for 5 minutes, count the flights you do and make a note so that you can compete with yourself.

There are many ideas around you that you can utilise to increase your movement and contribute to an exercise regime, which will help to:

increase metabolic rate;

increase energy expenditure;

build or maintain muscle mass;

support joint health too;

get more oxygen into your body and brain;

increase bodily movement, which is also good for the brain (keeping it nimble!);

boost your mood;

reduce risk of chronic diseases such as cancer, diabetes and heart disease;

improve your sex life;

act as a good de-stresser;

improve sleep.

All of this and it will help you to improve your weight management aims by having a great, toned figure. What more can you ask?

DON'T FORGET VITAMIN D3!

Vitamin D deficiency is very widespread and it's such a simple thing to rectify. It could be causing you problems with your general wellbeing that will become more evident if you start a diet regime. A 2009 study linked Vitamin D3 levels with weight loss success. Researchers found that pre-diet levels had a direct relationship to predicted weight loss and for each unit of measurement (ng/ml) of increase in Vitamin D levels, weight loss increased by up to half a pound without further modification to the diet regime. An additional benefit of a greater loss of abdominal fat was found with improved Vitamin D levels. But there are also some very important reasons why your Vitamin D level is important.

Vitamin D Deficiency - Serious Stuff

Vitamin D deficiency is linked with:

- Increased storage of fat around the middle;

- Decreased muscle mass;

- Increasing stress hormones that raise blood pressure;

- Increasing insulin resistance;

- Decreasing insulin release;

-Increasing inflammation in the body;

- Loss of bone mass, higher risk of cancer, autoimmune diseases and depression ...

So what does that mean to you?

More fat less muscle = more strain on your skeleton in terms of a bigger, heavier frame supported by less muscular leverage to carry you and a potential loss of bone mass or density, which means that your bones are not as solid and strong as they could be.

Increases in blood pressure and inflammation are very real markers and risk factors for heart disease, accelerating the ageing process.

The increase in insulin resistance and lowering of insulin release will increase your risk of diabetes or even put you in a pre-diabetic state. With diabetes, many health problems are escalated to a new level.

What is Vitamin D3?

This vitamin is more commonly known as the 'sunshine vitamin' and deficiency may have been enhanced by a fear of the sun (or skin cancers) and the over application of sunscreen. Your skin actually needs to go a bit pink in the sun and in the summer, allowing 15 – 30 minutes of exposure will do your D levels the power of good.

Vitamin D is really a hormone that is produced by the body when it is exposed to the right sort of UV sunlight. You can also get limited top ups from your diet and red meat and fish are the best foods but this route involves a metabolic process.

You have receptors for Vitamin D all around your body including the important hormones producing glands - thyroid, adrenals, ovaries/testes, thymus, pancreas and pituitary - as well as in your gut, nervous system (brain and spinal cord) and bones.

Factors That Can Increase Your Risk of D Deficiency

Darker Skin

If you have darker skin your need for Vitamin D is greater because dark skin means that it takes more exposure to sunlight for the body to be able to make it and therefore levels may be more depleted than a lighter skinned person.

Prescription and Over-The-Counter Drugs

Some prescription and OTC drugs can deplete your body's level of Vitamin D3:

Proton Pump Inhibitors such as omeprazole and ranitidine.

Antacids such as Tums (calcium carbonate) and Milk of Magnesia.

Some antibiotics.

Calcium Channel Blockers for high blood pressure such as amlodipine.

Statins - a sign may be that you are experiencing muscular aches and pains.

Steroids

And finally, weight loss drugs Fat Inhibitors such as Alli and Xenical.

Getting a simple test can help you establish where your level is, which is an important step in taking your Vitamin D level serious and also moving towards a better health profile.

THE NEED FOR RELAXATION

We live in a 24 hour, 7 day week society. We always seem to be connected to someone, virtually. We don't get time to be quiet and just be with those people in our immediate environment or on our own. Communication expectations are immense both at work and at home – texting, social networks, Skype/Facetime, emails, phone calls …. This is but one factor of our 21st century lives that can contribute significantly to stress.

If stress is tension and closed, relaxation is loose and open. Openness is a more accepting state, less controlling and is more creative; whereas, stress and tension means more cortisol, which inhibits cognitive function and shrinks your hippocampus (your brain's memory centre).

Relaxation is very important for a positive sense of wellbeing and if you have a positive sense of wellbeing you are more likely to make good choices and decisions for yourself – including diet and exercise. This is perhaps more important than you realise because many people start diets and most fail with their aims of long term weight loss and body shape change never getting off the ground floor. Why? Because they don't give themselves the space, mental and emotional, to make the behavioural changes that are needed, as well as the important change in mindset about how to see themself as a reflection in their own mirror. This change in mindset is all part of believing in your success and knowing that once you've achieved it, you will maintain it. This clarity of vision will help you to overcome the habits, or subconscious drivers, of the 3 E's (because the biochemical drivers, your hormones, have been quietened through better understanding), not just in the short term, but permanently.

Relaxing?

How do you relax? In front of the tv? With a glass of wine and something to nibble? Do you have your phone by your side so that you can keep up with your friends on Facebook, listen for texts and emails?

This is not relaxation. This is distraction. Distraction is a behaviour that has been developed to make up for relaxation. The trouble is that distraction is tiring and it's all about keeping yourself entertained, to avoid thinking about things in your life, planning or organising any form of personal development and, yes, that includes successful weight management, in a way that is health-giving and sustaining rather than purely convenient. Convenient weight loss products surround us at the supermarket and the pharmacy and yet they are just another way of distracting yourself (at financial cost) from the real issue, which is looking after yourself in a positive and nourishing way – physically, mentally and emotionally.

Top Tips for Relaxing

1   Make it a sensory experience:

Massage (with your partner or book yourself for a regular treat)

Facial/beauty treatment (exchange with a friend or book a regular treat)

Breakfast in bed on a Sunday – have a relaxing special breakfast of fresh fruit and yoghurt or cold meat and cheese with a herbal tea.

Go for a walk! The weather doesn't matter, it's part of the sensory experience. If it's raining and windy wrap up and go out, so what if you're going to get wet and buffeted about - enjoy it! Laugh; and, then come home and have a hot bath or shower and a nice cup of tea.

2   Transport yourself somewhere else:

Read a novel - it's a great way to take yourself off into a different world that can completely engulf you and help you to let go of stresses and strains on all levels.

Watch a movie - there are a number of online options where you can select something to transport you to that different world. No distractions ... no food or phones, get lost in the story.

3   Music

Music can be very evocative, stirring emotion that may have been buried, but it can also help to change your mood more positively. Studies have shown that a decrease in blood pressure, a drop in cortisol, and relief from anxiety and pain can all be achieved through music therapy and this is something we can use so easily in our everyday lives. Choose well.

4   Meditation and Mindfulness

There are around 2500 studies that have been published on meditation and how it can benefit your wellbeing. It can be a little intimidating to those who have never tried it, but there are many techniques that can lead you towards a meditative state. An excellent one to start with is just coming into the present moment whenever and wherever you are. Coming into the present with your whole mind and awareness is a way of not only quietening the continual buzz of mind chatter but also of becoming more perceptive about what's going on around you in the present moment. It can even help you to improve your concentration and focus. This is the practice of mindfulness. Mindfulness is a powerful reminder that we only have each moment by moment in which to truly live life. Try this exercise ...

Next time you make yourself a cup of tea stop for a moment. Focus on what you are doing: choose a cup from the cupboard that is a comfortable or special cup to you, not the chipped one that just comes to hand because it's there. As you fill the kettle be aware and grateful that the water that comes out of your tap is clean and abundant. Consciously choose your tea and get the milk from the fridge, appreciating each movement and thought, conscious and unconscious, as you move across the room. Make your tea and sit for a moment, look at your tea, feel its warmth and smell it. As you sip from your favourite cup appreciate the tea's flavour and just sit for a moment and enjoy. This is a practice that you can do discreetly wherever and whenever - it will bring you into the moment and help you to appreciate what you do eat and drink through your day. You might find that it's the most satisfying cup of tea that you've had in years!

5   Love

Feeling loved and loving someone back is one of the best de-stressors of all and there is hard scientific evidence that love and meaningful friendships will support your health and wellbeing. If you have any doubts about this you might want to check out James Lynch's book, *A Cry Unheard: New Insights into Medical Consequences of Loneliness*, which goes into many aspects of loneliness and how profoundly it affects our health.

Love helps you to feel connected and in feeling connected you feel supported and understood, which helps you to   make better choices about how you look after yourself because you feel valued.

MORE TIPS & TRICKS FOR WEIGHT LOSS

What are You Feeding Your Mind?

Being conscious and selective about what you expose yourself to may be a new concept for you. But stop and think how much input during your day stresses you, saddens you, offends you, makes you angry or anxious?

Increased awareness about your daily life will help you to create change for the better.

Input Audit

What TV and Film Genres Do You Watch?

Question to Self: am I watching negative programmes to make my life look better whilst, as the credits roll, realising that I feel quite depressed or frustrated?

Action

Be selective and watch programmes that inspire or educate, giving you positive energy for life and living.

How Are You With Your Friends and Family and How Are They With You?

Question to Self: are my friends dramas bringing me down? Am I being constantly drained by family and friends for advice and support, leaving nothing for me?

Action

Assess your relationships and, if necessary, put some distance between you and those who drain you List the people in your life who are important and start it with yourself! *You have to be selfish in order to be selfless.* This is a concept that many women, in particular, struggle with as mums and carers, but you have to look after yourself and your needs first, in order to look after children and be there for others. Take yourself seriously and give yourself permission.

How Many Forms of Contact Are You Available Through? How Available Are You?

Question to Self: how much do I allow myself to be at the beck and call of my phone, emails or my social network? Are other people setting the agenda for my life?

Action

Turn off ... yes, turn off, your phone and computer after a certain point in your evening. Make it a ground rule that in order to spend real time with yourself and those in your immediate environment you only have your contact points open until 8pm or 9pm and then that's it until 8am next morning. This will help you to feel more connected, instead of less connected, to the people in your real life over those in your virtual life. Sharing your life more fully with those around you can bring you much needed support and encouragement when your aims are to make positive lifestyle changes.

Are there other areas of your life that you would like to make changes?

Start with your daily routine and make small changes – they are much more realistic and sustainable.

Once you feel confident about your daily routine start to

look at some of the bigger issues and tackle them one by one – be kind to you and to others. It doesn't have to be harsh and challenging. Bringing awareness into your daily living will help you to make better and better choices about what influences you want in your life as well as how you treat yourself.

Mindfulness

Mindfulness is something we discussed in *The Need for Relaxation* as it helps to create a more relaxed and open feeling. It is a singular form of awareness that helps you to stay in the present, rather than get wrapped up in thought processes about the past or the future. Stressful thoughts about the past and present will enhance negative emotions that could have you indulging in one or more of the 3 E's again! Mindfulness is a form of awake meditation that helps you to be more open and accepting of your life as it is happening. This is nothing like being self-conscious, which is closed and judging.

I highly recommend finding out more about mindfulness practice.

Look at Your Food Budget

A change in diet and lifestyle often means new substitute or 'slimming' foods, equipment for the kitchen, visits to the health shop and many other ways in which to introduce expense and stress around adopting a more healthy lifestyle. But it doesn't have to be that way.

Try IF

Intermittent Fasting is an effective and simple way to integrate a weight loss or management regime that will actually cut your food budget, not make your life more expensive or complicated.

Here are some things I really like about IF:

- It's simple, you just stop eating for a few hours - biological markers that relate to ill-health and chronic disease will change for the better.

- It saves you money and gives you time that you would otherwise spend on preparing and eating food.

You can still have the 'yummy' stuff.

- It works with a social life. If you go out for a meal with friends you can change your fast day, or, if you have a particularly hard day gardening or travelling, move your fast day to another day in the week (never fast after a lot of stress or exertion).

Your metabolism likes variety of input!

Eat Breakfast Like a King, Lunch Like a Prince and Dinner Like a Pauper

A new study (2013) suggests that the timing of your meals can make a big difference to weight loss progress. It was a small study that put two groups of women on the same diet of three meals of 700 calories, 500 and 200 (1400 calories in total). Half of the women had the larger meal in the morning for breakfast (700 calories) with 200 in the evening and the other half had the small breakfast with a larger meal in the evening. The larger meal even included a bar of chocolate or desert. Over the twelve week period that the diet was followed the women who had the larger meal for breakfast lost 8.7 kg (over 19 lbs), whilst the other group lost 5.1 kg (over 11 lbs).

This study presents a new perspective on dieting as it takes into account the body's ability to use energy though the day as part of your daily calorie consumption. It makes sense to have a good meal to set yourself up for the day, unfortunately it's the one we tend to give less emphasis to. For most people running out of the door first thing in the morning to get to work, or the children to school, tends to be more important than sitting down and spending some time getting your metabolic fire going for the day ahead.

Food for thought?

Eating Consciously

How many times do you eat something without paying attention and then wish there was more?

How many times do you eat or drink something and then wish you hadn't?

Action

Create ground rules of respect. Respect for what you put into your body as well as respect for yourself.

Do you want to use your stomach as a rubbish bin? Go for quality because yes, you're worth it!

Only eat when you can sit and really take notice of, and enjoy, the food you put in your mouth. Don't do what I witnessed on the London Underground recently – I watched a young woman standing in a crowded carriage literally stuffing a boxed salad, mouthful by mouthful, whilst balancing heavy bags in the moving train. What is the point? It was unpleasant to witness and revealed a possible fear about missing a meal. Intermittent Fasting will help to overcome that myth – you won't starve and fall over!

Eat only when you can do it properly - make this a firm rule and it will automatically take out wasteful and unconscious snacking. You will also find that as you appreciate each mouthful and its flavour and texture your stomach recognises that it is being fed much more quickly and this will help your body recognise satiety (feeling full or satisfied) much more quickly and allow you a better understanding of your need regarding portion control.

Keep a food diary. This is not for anyone but you to record your intake – note everything! Drinks, snacks, meals – when and where. You might be shocked at how much you consume in a day. Honesty might be harsh but it's the only way to recognise weak points and cravings, as well as the quantity and quality of your diet.

Look at what you are doing and plan ahead.

Easi-Tips

If you drink wine, perhaps to a bit of excess and find it hard to say no once you've opened the bottle …

either: buy a more expensive wine that makes you stop and savour what you have bought. *Less is more.*

Or: buy a soda water or sparkling water and make spritzers, half and half, to fool yourself that you are drinking more. *More is less.*

If you're a coffee addict there's a strategy I recommend to help to wean yourself off dependency.

Set a rule that you have no coffee after 1pm. (This may help with disrupted sleep patterns too!)

If you have 4 coffees in the morning make the last one a decaffeinated. Do that for a week and then reduce to three. Give yourself a week and reduce again.

Find a good organic coffee and if you use ground or filter coffee, make the transition using the principles above and migrate to an instant coffee.

You can also make your coffee using half caffeinated and half decaffeinated.

Keep your coffee treats, like Lattes, for when you go out – maybe at the weekend. It's so much more scrummy!

Do you suffer with a willpower lapse when it comes to sugar cravings?

Keeping your blood sugar levels under control is important, not only for dieting but also for your health and wellbeing. Living with sugar cravings can make you a higher risk for diabetes.

Don't forget your metabolic fire! Think of your metabolism as a fire that needs feeding. If you throw a piece of paper on your fire, whoosh and it's gone in a quick blaze of glory, just like putting carbs (chocolate, cake, biscuits, crisps, etc) into your stomach, it raises your blood sugar quickly and then crashes to nothing, leaving you feeling worse than you did before. But if you put some protein into your stomach (some nuts, quality whey protein, some organic chicken for example) you are putting the equivalent of a log on your metabolic fire. It will be a slow burn, releasing energy steadily in a sustained fashion that won't have you flying on the ceiling and then crashing and burning.

There's a trick I recommend for providing a more sustained energy level:

Use a good quality whey protein shake that contains essential amino acids. (Amino acids are the individual building blocks of your peptides (short chain proteins) and proteins that help to maintain and repair your body.) You can use it as a snack support during the day by putting a scoop into some yoghurt or cold milk with ice and a banana. Or, you can use it as a meal replacement by using two scoops in a protein shake with fruit and milk. This goes back to our metabolic fire explained earlier in the book and helps to sustain your energy levels more solidly than topping up on simple carbs.

If you find that mornings are hard to get through then look at having a protein based breakfast of eggs for example, or perhaps go continental and have cold meal and cheese.

Keep Your Fluids Up!

Your body is about 75% water, keeping your fluids up will help you to keep your brain awake and you won't be driven to overeat when you are actually thirsty.

Your body needs water and the early sensations of hunger and thirst are very similar and easily mistaken.

Another useful pointer with regard to weight loss comes from Dr Batmanghelidj in his book, *Obesity, Cancer, Depression: Their Common Cause and Natural Cure*:

> "Taking a glass of water before eating would also stimulate secretion of [the hormones]adrenaline and noradrenaline by the sympathetic nervous system for at least two hours. This direct action of

water on the sympathetic nervous system forcefully activates hormone-sensitive lipase to break down fat for use as energy to enhance the physical activity of the body. This is the reason water overrides the sensation of hunger in a short period of time."

Making the Shift With Your Self-Image

Are you someone who was always told that you were "chunky", "chubby", "well-covered", "flabby" or plain "fat" – words to that effect? Or, is it that since the children were born your pre-pregnancy shape disappeared never to be seen again. You don't like it but it happens to most women, right? Well, no, not really.

If these ideas, or ones like them, have become adopted by you as an unchangeable feature of who you are, you are setting yourself up for being a continual failure at losing weight. Self-image is an important aspect of success and you really need to engage with a vision of yourself as a slimmer, more toned and happy version of yourself, bearing in mind that you have also massively reduced the risk factors for chronic diseases along the way. This should make you feel very happy and positive about your health and wellbeing.

In the words of William Anderson, who devised *The Anderson Method: the secret to permanent weight loss is to change your self-image:*

> *"Want to live the rest of your life at a healthy weight? Start here: Spend a little time each day thinking about it, imagining yourself fit at the weight you want to be. Picture how you'll look, what you'll do, what you'll wear. Daydream about yourself in the clothes you'd like, being active, feeling good, living life at your target weight. Imagine yourself at all the ages of your life that are coming, lean and fit and happy in all of them. Picture yourself eating healthfully, enjoying the foods you like in healthy amounts, easily able to maintain self-control and moderation."*

In order to be successful you must believe that you will be. Create your vision and be that vision. Find images of someone who could be your role model, create your vision board or page in your notebook, use quotes to motivate and inspire yourself. Work it, mould it and ultimately be it!

Supplemental Help

5-HTP

5-HTP (L-5-hydroxytryptophan) - is a dietary supplement from the seeds of the Griffonia plant and is a precursor, or building block of serotonin. It can support the production of serotonin and melatonin, helping to balance mood, sleep cycles and appetite. 5-HTP has been studied to show that it is more effective than Prozac in its ability to support people through depression and anxiety.

Recommended dose - 100-600 mg

NB 5-HTP should not be taken with anti-depressants, weight control drugs or other serotonin modifying drugs or substances known to cause liver damage. People with compromised liver function may not be able to regulate 5-HTP properly.

GABA

A little known food supplement that is a major inhibitory neurotransmitter, GABA (Gamma-Aminobutyric Acid) helps to prevent the over-firing of nerve cells by blocking the transmission of an impulse from one cell to another. This is how GABA can help to promote a greater sense of relaxation in people who are over-anxious or agitated. It can also help to promote sleep.

It could be used as an alternative to reaching for alcohol in the evenings, to help you unwind, rest and relax, which can help you to manage your mood and energy levels.

Recommended dosage 300-750 mg three times per day.

NB People with liver or kidney disease should check with their doctor before using GABA.

Multi Vitamin and Mineral

I believe that it is always worth supplementing your diet with a high quality multi vitamin and mineral product, which can help to address nutritional deficiencies through poor dietary choices as well as restrictive calorie regimes. A good product will provide support for your adrenals and thyroid function.

IS ADVANCED HORMONE TESTING FOR YOU?

Conventional medical practice uses blood testing to look at steroid (fat-based) hormones such as oestrogen, progesterone, testosterone, DHEAS and cortisol, but the hormone level seen in blood is bound to a carrier protein making it unavailable to its target tissues. In other words it doesn't do anything. It's only the unbound fraction, about 1-5%, that is available to move into the receptors and make the many connections that these amazing biochemical messengers make. This active level of hormone is what we need to know about because it's directly related to whether you will experience symptoms of hormone excess or deficiency, which may be adversely affecting your wellbeing and influencing your potential health risk factors.

We need to remember that doctors are most interested in signs of disease and many hormone imbalances can adversely affect your wellbeing and quality of life without signs or problems of disease. However, if these signs are left unattended they may become more significant health issues such as diabetes, high blood pressure, obesity, depression and many others.

I work with advanced hormone testing through saliva, which is able to provide us with levels of the active hormone. This can be a very revealing process that ultimately makes so much sense to the individual. We look at adrenal function because it can tell us so many things about why an individual may be experiencing: poor sleep, susceptibility to allergies and autoimmune issues, weight gain around the middle, depression, anxiety, infertility, memory and thinking problems. Adrenal health is an area that medicine mostly sidelines and yet poor function here can have a profound influence on so many levels of your wellbeing.

The secret of hormone health is to view it through the experience of the individual and to join the dots of data you can collate to make a very revealing picture about the many symptoms they may be experiencing. Many long standing health issues can simply disappear: hay fever, IBS, weight management, depression … It's all about supporting the network as naturally as possible so that your body (the most complex biochemical factory that is beyond man's imagination) can begin to re-orchestrate its own symphony. This is not a claim that hormone health will magically or successfully address all ills but it can help you to understand and work with your body more successfully to maintain good health and wellbeing through the ageing process we call life.

Having read this book you are now much more aware of the broad impacts of your hormone health on your weight and your ability to control it, but if you want some real data to work with advanced hormone testing might be for you.

There's a Weight Management Profile

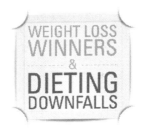

Weight Management Profile
Clinical Quality Testing Made Simple

This advanced hormone test can be done at home and can look at hormones that have very specific relationships to weight management issues, which might be getting in the way of your healthy intentions to lose weight and reduce your risk factors for a number of degenerative diseases, such as diabetes and heart disease.

What Hormones Does It Test?

Oestrogen and Progesterone Balance - this is important for men and women because excess Oestrogen from the Pill or HRT for women and extra weight for men and women is linked with ongoing problems such as: weight gain at the hips and breasts (this can be especially noticeable for men with moobs or man-boobs); water retention, mood as well as affecting thyroid hormone availability.

Testosterone and DHEA - this is another area that can have direct impact on energy levels and ability to motivate and exercise because chronically low levels will cause or contribute to: decreased muscle mass, a lower metabolic rate and central obesity, or fat around the middle!

Cortisol - stress profile - cortisol issues can increase appetite, causing sugar cravings and low energy levels by inhibiting thyroid hormones that control your metabolism.

Vitamin D3 - a deficiency in this important vitamin may be behind insulin resistance, increased abdominal fat and mood issues.

TSH - otherwise known as Thyroid Stimulating Hormone - is a primary test for thyroid gland dysfunction. It won't give a complete view of thyroid hormone issues but it does let us know if your pituitary is 'shouting' at your thyroid because it's not producing enough thyroid hormone.

Fasting Insulin and HbA1c - you couldn't have a better profile to identify a pre-diabetic or diabetic state that hasn't previously been diagnosed and requires some serious attention. If it is previously undiagnosed it is most likely that sensible changes to your diet and lifestyle, bringing weight reduction will reverse any problems.

Your test results come with an explanatory report - it's not just lab results! So you can really start to learn where your Dieting Downfalls are so that you can work to overcome them instead of having them sabotage your efforts and willpower time and time again.

Standard medical healthcare approaches don't always have all the answers. They are able to treat you with medicines but there is a great deal that you can do for yourself to improve your wellbeing and your long-term health so that you can look forward to a happy, healthy older age.

CONCLUDING THOUGHTS

Losing weight and managing your lifestyle for your wellbeing can be challenging in our 24/7 world that's geared towards convenience and solutions-in-a-box that promise results without real effort. But first, think about your health – does this convenience work in your best interests?

Many people think that their doctor will sort them out if it all goes too wrong. Doctors don't have all the answers. Drugs and surgery are not the answer when it comes to a weight problem or the prevention of the chronic diseases associated with it: diabetes, coronary heart disease and cancer, to name a few. Drugs don't cure diseases, they manage symptoms and potentially create side effects that can be very uncomfortable to live with. Medicine cannot continue to dig us out of the hole of neglect and abuse, we have to be responsible for taking better care of ourselves.

The Weight Loss Voyage on a Sea of Change

The information in this book aims to help you to make significant steps on your own weight loss voyage. There are tips and tricks that you can use to make the baby steps you need to make, so that the changes you choose are permanent, not temporary and easily defeated.

Here are the stages for you to transition through...

Identify what you want to *BECOME*

Your realistic ideal weight;
Your realistic ideal dress or trouser size;
Exercise aims and schedule;
What are your motivators?
Find a picture of yourself or a role model to remind you of your vision.

Do you believe what you have said above? Honestly, to the bottom of your heart?

Identify the qualities of *BEING* that person

Understanding your motivators - have you found that they have changed or do you just understand yourself better?

Personal disciplines:
    Exercise;
    Willpower;
    Diet;
    Sleep;
    Are you feeding your mind with the right material?

What are the benefits you are experiencing?

Your personal development:
    Self-responsibility;
    Self-confidence;
    Sense of achievement.

Maintaining *YOUR LIFESTYLE*

Continuing to shape and refine your personal dietary guidelines.

Exploring your personal disciplines and looking at the benefits of:
    The social;
    The physical;
    The mental;
    The emotional.

How is your confidence growing and shaping your life?

Is there a new job or promotion?

Are your health risk factors minimised?

Are you enjoying a new wardrobe of clothes?

Is your special relationship more intimate and fulfilling?

Work with yourself on the holistic and personal level and your voyage into weight loss on the sea of change will truly bring you to a new destination rather than back to the port from which you started.

Good luck and be healthy – always.

Recommended Reading

A Cry Unheard: New Insights into the medical consequences of loneliness –
James J Lynch

Excitotoxins: the taste that kills –
Russell Blaylock

Obesity, Cancer, Depression: their common cause and natural cure –
Dr F Batmanghelidj

The Anderson Method –
William Anderson

The End of Stress as We Know It –
Bruce McEwen

The Fast Diet: the simple secret of intermittent fasting –
Dr Michael Mosley and Mimi Spencer

It would be great if you could leave me an online review! There are so many diets that people try, if you think that the information in this book has helped you to understand why you might have had problems in the past when it comes to dieting please let others know! These lovely people emailed me directly …

I found it very illuminating and a great easy to read style. I can now see why some of the things I was doing previously were well intentioned but totally counterproductive! Janice, UK

I think it's a great angle in the dieting debate. I found it very readable and accessible with clear explanations. This is where your book comes in with its strategies for success and help to avoid the pitfalls. I think that it is very helpful not to be told that the reasons for self sabotage are all psychological – childhood baggage, but your hormones also play a large part in your body's lack of response. Dora, UK

I've bought the book and am half way through it. It is great, very, very clear. Debbie, UK

We have both read your book whilst we've been away and found it fascinating. Susan & Jeremy, UK

I thoroughly enjoyed reading your book. It was very informative and made so much sense.   Sharon, UK

ABOUT THE AUTHOR

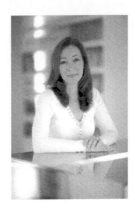

Dr Alyssa Burns-Hill, PhD, MSc, FRSPH, MIHPE is an international Hormone & Holistic Health Specialist with clinics in Harley Street, London and the Lido Medical Centre, Jersey. She also runs a virtual clinic with clients as far afield as Australia, Canada, Singapore, Brazil and Greece as well as all over the UK. She is the hormone health expert for the CMA (Complementary Medical Association), and is on the Advisory Panel for Thyroid UK.

Alyssa works with state-of-the-art hormone testing and uses her knowledge of hormone health to provide advanced analysis of often complex health scenarios.

Her unique approach is holistic and treats the whole person, because hormones affect us physically, mentally and emotionally. She empowers her clients to understand their own health better.

Alyssa's background in health stretches over 20 years and includes other published books and articles as well as national TV appearances.

www.dralyssaburns-hill.com

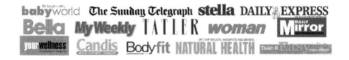

Printed in Great Britain
by Amazon.co.uk, Ltd.,
Marston Gate.